STRONG MOTHERS

MORE THAN A SURVIVAL GUIDE

CHRISTINA MORRIS

FEATURING: PAT BELL, ARICKA BRAZER, LAURA DI FRANCO, JACQUELINE M. KANE, KANDI LEIGH, ALI LEVINE, LISA LICKERT, SALLY MARTIN, LAURA MCKINNON, ANGELA MEDWAY SMITH, LINDA AILEEN MILLER, LAYNE ELIESE MILLS, DR. PAMELA J. PINE, DR. AHRIANA PLATTEN, LISA RUSSEL, TANYA SAUNDERS, MICHELE TATOS, LULU TREVENA, ATLANTIS WOLF

STRONG
MOTHERS

MORE THAN A SURVIVAL GUIDE

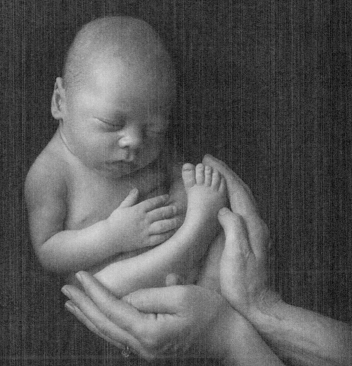

CHRISTINA MORRIS

FEATURING: PAT BELL, ARICKA BRAZER, LAURA DI FRANCO, JACQUELINE M KANE, KANDI LEIGH, ALI LEVINE, LISA LICKERT, SALLY MARTIN, LAURA MCKINNON, ANGELA MEDWAY SMITH, LINDA AILEEN MILLER, LAYNE ELIESE MILLS, DR. PAMELA J. PINE, DR. AHRIANA PLATTEN, LISA RUSSELL, TANYA SAUNDERS, MICHELE TATOS, LULU TREVENA, ATLANTIS WOLF

DEDICATION

From the bottom of my heart, I thank my beautiful boy,
who has inspired me beyond belief. I'm grateful to you every day.

To my husband for always being my biggest supporter
and for giving me the gift of motherhood.

To the amazing women in this book,
thank you for your bravery in sharing your powerful stories.
The gift of your encouraging words to the world
can help heal wounds and open doors that were previously closed.

To all my wonderful friends and family,
I'm lucky to have my amazing circle,
and I appreciate you all even more after experiencing isolation.

Thank you to you, dear reader. If you're a mother or if you support mothers,
I hope this book gives you strength. I feel privileged you've picked up this book.
Here's to your healing journey.

DISCLAIMER:

This book offers health and nutritional information and is designed for educational purposes only. You should not rely on this information as a substitute for, nor does it replace professional medical advice, diagnosis, or treatment. If you have any concerns or questions about your health, you should always consult with a physician or other healthcare professional. Do not disregard, avoid, or delay obtaining medical or health-related advice from your healthcare professional because of something you may have read here. The use of any information provided in this book is solely at your own risk.

Developments in medical research may impact the health, fitness, and nutritional advice that appears here. No assurances can be given that the information contained in this book will always include the most relevant findings or developments with respect to the particular material.

Having said all that, know that the experts here have shared their tools, practices, and knowledge with you with a sincere and generous intent to assist you on your health and wellness journey. Please contact them with any questions you may have about the techniques or information they provided. They will be happy to assist you further!

TABLE OF CONTENTS

INTRODUCTION

*"Every problem that humans experience
is born from the illusion of separate self."*

- Deepak Chopra

Some life experiences shock us into enlightenment - we can contribute more to this world than we already have. My pregnancy was certainly one of those adventures, but it was how I handled a particular incident afterwards that made me see how much I had strengthened myself during pregnancy. I knew then that this book needed to be written, and these tools needed to be shared.

It was a beautiful sunny day, the type when the sun fills you from your toes to the top of your head with a warm, fuzzy feeling. My son was an early arrival, and it wasn't lost on me that, in a parallel existence, I should have been sitting in my cold, dismal home office. I soaked in the sunbeams dancing on my face in the crisp air.

My baby boy was becoming restless. On entry to the park, there was an old, wooden picnic bench with our name on it. I pulled my boy to me to feed him. I admired him as he fed. His skin was so silken and creamy like milky quartz. Little flecks of his hair started to show through on his head, but it was unclear if they were chocolate or auburn hairs just yet. He was only a newborn, and I only occasionally saw his sapphire eyes when he opened them. He often looked to be in hibernation, getting out into the big, bright world. His hands clasped at me. They were so soft and dainty, musician's hands with long, elegant fingers. Perhaps one day, he would play instruments, like his dad. His eyes started to flicker, his beautiful eyelashes like butterfly wings batting together. I soon noticed he was flicking his eyes because the sun was in his face. I swung my legs around the picnic bench and transferred us both to the other side—not knowing how pivotable this change would be.

He has settled again and was happy feeding. I looked up from him momentarily; I heard the noise. A Jeep smashed through the car park fence and accelerated towards us. I don't remember doing it, but I must have leaped from the bench at super speed because I only partially felt the impact. A woman got out of the vehicle. She must have been in shock herself because she selfishly exclaimed, "My car, my car!" She looked at my son and me as though we were ghosts or shadows. I felt dazed. Just then, a lovely woman came running towards me. She had blonde hair, light eyelashes, and a kind, freckled face. She said, "Oh my God! Are you all right?" She yelled something at the driver and proceeded to take us both to safety.

The incident showed me the kindness of strangers and how lucky we were. We moved from the other side of the bench moments before the crash. It was as though my boy told me to move. He blinked dramatically because of the light, and that saved us from being seriously injured or, for him, worse.

This accident could have freaked any new mum out on their first long walk, alone since giving birth, but I believe because I had already put so many tools in place during pregnancy to make me strong, I was resilient when it happened. This confirmed the need for this book; to share the tools I learned and the tools from other amazing mothers (biological mothers, adoptive mothers, doulas, and mothers of communities).

Here is our guide so that you can be a strong mother when the time comes.

CHAPTER 1

A MOTHER IS BORN

TURNING PREGNANCY CHALLENGES INTO TRANSFORMATION

Christina Morris

MY STORY

I run my index finger down his forehead and nose. My hands are paler than usual due to the cool English weather. Next to his unweathered, alabaster skin and the coral polish adorning my nails, my fingers appear to glow. I stroke his nose repeatedly. On close inspection, a soft, silken peach fuzz of fur glides over it. His nose slopes gently like mine. I have a memory of my mum doing the same on my ski-slope nose. "Soft and squishy like a piece of putty," she would say.

The sunlight dances through the burnt orange curtains left by the previous owners, and a warm clementine haze highlights the room. He throws his pudgy arms up in the air resembling a flamenco dancer. It startles me, and I think I've woken him. He's still sleeping. He places his hands in a dramatic pose creating a frame around his face. *How can his hands be comfortable when flexed like that?* But he is comfortable, blissfully so. If you told me in the previous months that I would be content watching my baby sleep in a suburban house that we now call home, I wouldn't have believed you, but I am content, blissfully so.

I felt like a baby myself—a newborn ripped from the womb and placed on a clinical metal slab under white, bleaching lights, vulnerable and confused. They say it takes a village to raise a child. So to have my entire tribe of loved ones severed from me during my first pregnancy due to the pandemic isolation rules left me blindsided. Yes, I'd chosen to live in London, but it was always reassuring to know my family was only five hours away. This reassurance was obsolete in a pandemic.

"Higher, higher. To the left," my mum said as I tried to show her my baby bump on a video call. "Maybe, down a bit," my friend said, followed by, "You know what? Maybe send me a photo."

The pandemic isolation will lift, and I'll be able to hug everyone, and they can feel my pregnancy bump. I kept telling myself. *I can't wait for all my family to be together at Christmas.* These are the pipe dreams that kept me going. I didn't get the chance to hug everyone, and Christmas was canceled. We were legally not allowed to leave our homes.

It wasn't only this that was difficult during my pregnancy. For the six months previous, I was in my lonely apartment every day, as my husband was able to leave the house. I always enjoy meeting people and bouncing ideas off one another. The office in my old apartment looked out onto a dark alleyway, except it didn't look out; the glass was frosted. Sometimes the highlight of my day was a local cat who came and sat on the ledge. I watched his elegant silhouette licking his paws and looking into the window as though he wanted to offer me empathetic comfort. It reminded me of learning about Plato's Cave in high school ethics class—that most people see only shadows of the world. I knew there was more beyond that shadow, and I was desperate to get out. I was like a sunflower without light, and we all know what happens to plants without enough light: they wilt.

Throughout my life, I was always excited to be a mother, but strangely the closer I got to it, the more I would say, "Just a few more years." Being happily married, I was open to growing our family but not just yet. However, my body and the universe had other ideas.

I started to feel inadequate and questioned myself. *Maybe I didn't want to be a mother? Had I always wanted this?* I even started to hear the unwelcome opinion of the anxious part of my brain; *You probably won't be a good mum.* These feelings sat on me, they were a paperweight trapping a sheet of parchment from the wind. I tried to lift them.

My pregnancy experience with my loved ones was stolen from me and it felt like rock salt in an open wound. None of my family members or friends experienced my growing bump. None of them felt the kicks become stronger. I think it was because of this sadness that I felt massively intimidated by motherhood.

I'm so glad I journaled all of this at the time because I was so cruel to myself. Looking back on it now, I am, like everyone, an imperfect human being, but at my core, I've always had a kind heart, and surely someone with an open heart cannot be destined to be a truly awful mum.

I didn't know that these cruel thoughts affect millions of pregnant women. The hormonal imbalance coursed through my veins like molten lava. I had heard of women's postnatal struggles, never prenatal, and because of my lack of awareness, I assumed this was just my genuine thought process, and I wholeheartedly believed my mean thoughts about myself.

The screen and my dank office became too much, so I booked a week off work. I drove to the seaside. The chalky rock face of the English coastline was looking onto the sea and seemed serene on this particular day. The autumn sun glimmered across the water like glass or a precious gem. Growing up next to a beach has always made me love the coast. It has always calmed me. I associate the water with tranquillity and enjoy nature's meditative soundtrack of the ocean waves. I walked along the edge of the precipice, my rubber wellie boots traipsing through the marram grass. I pulled my thick faux fur coat tighter around me to brace the wind. The seagrass across the chalk rock looked like tufts of hair on a baby's bald head. I walked to the furthest point I could. The ground was uneven underfoot.

I hit a wall, and something had to change. I stood there, looking out at the expansive sea, but it was like I couldn't see anything at all. I thought horrible thoughts about myself. A huge cloud and shadow reigned over me.

The salty air caressed my hair and my face as I stood in silence. I was sure I felt movement in my stomach, but it was far too early in the pregnancy for that. It was as though he whispered to me, "It's going to be okay." I listened.

Getting back in my car, tears and the saline wind had left my face stinging. This day was a catalyst. I promised myself there and then that I would get myself better and not only be a good mum, but become the best mum I could be.

I'd always had a negative mindset. I used to tell myself things wouldn't happen so I would be pleasantly surprised if they did. After my turning point on the beach, I spent the following months educating myself on positive mentality and therapeutic actions. I enjoyed life coaching courses, an amazing self-development book club, and lots of additional reading to get myself to where I wanted to be.

Every morning, I woke up early and journaled about what I was grateful for. I bought a diary on a trip to Devon in early pregnancy—a child's book, bright yellow and complete with a lock and "Be Happy" emblazoned across the garish front cover. At the time, that slogan made me eye-roll heavily. I remember feeling infuriated that the only diary I could find in the quaint market town of Totnes was from a large bookstore chain rather than a local gift shop, but I needed it, and, boy, am I glad I bought it. I didn't know the impact those lined pages would have. I forced myself to write ten different gratitudes every day. Something about the pen to the page made the thankfulness more real.

I would sit and meditate every day on what I was grateful for, using breathwork I learned from meditation courses and years of martial arts, and new techniques from virtual pregnancy yoga and hypno-birthing doula classes. I would breathe in positivity and breathe out negative thoughts.

One of the biggest shifts in my mindset was my gratitude for my ability to exercise in nature. I already started cycling to overcome the dreariness of being locked down in the four walls of my office, but questioned if I should continue through pregnancy. I did. I cycled throughout the entirety of my pregnancy, and I'm so glad I did. The rides became shorter and I avoided the hills as time went on, but I went every day religiously. I rode each day through the fascinating landscape where we lived at the time—nature woven into the synthetic. Many would think this route was dismal, but I was grateful for the smallest of things; I saw it as a chaotic beauty. Swans and geese adjusted to their man-made surroundings, gliding along the reservoir and canals. The wheels of my bicycle turned alongside the birds drifting through the algae waters. The horse paddocks and fields I rode past had the industrial factory of a bakery looming over them, and yet there was so much greenery and breathing space; the smell of baked goods and nature were amalgamated and co-existing. Even in a dense city, connecting with nature helped soothe my mind and soul and was, in itself, a meditation.

My baby would often kick excitedly as I cycled. Knowing my child was a boy bonded me to him in a way I can't explain. I always pictured my firstborn being a boy. *It* was a he now, a him, a person, and I would think about him a lot. *What would he look like? How would he be?* I started to get excited about being a mum, and I believe getting to know *him* helped.

I'm happy to say I loved my son from the moment I first met him in the world. But I believe all my actions in pregnancy helped me get to that place. I was worried that wouldn't be the case, as many are unable to shift their mindset.

My son had issues with his heartbeat the week prior to his birth, and I went to the hospital worried, but they checked and told me he would be fine.

It was early morning, I had sleep taste in my mouth, and I felt the warm trickle of liquid on my legs. I stood, waiting for this to turn into contractions, and a gush of fluid came instead. *The midwife told me this only happened in the movies.* I confusedly nudged my husband awake to say, "I think my waters have broken, but I'm not having contractions." After a call to the hospital, we were there half an hour later at 4 am. They said I could go home, but I felt uneasy. I hadn't felt his heartbeat for a while. I remember the disinfectant smell as I chatted in the clinically stark-white midwife's office, and the disconnect as my husband wasn't allowed to accompany me due to the virus. The midwife was a tired, abrupt woman who had little patience for my lack of contractions, and I was glad to be rid of her as she discharged me.

When I started to leave the hospital at 5 am, I felt dizzy. I asked my husband to come with me into the bathroom to help. He was not meant to be in there because of Covid, but I needed him. I sat on the floor, the bright, white light stinging my eyes. I felt a desire to be in a dark place, warm and comforted. My doula taught me that I would need a place like this during birth, so I knew my little boy was on his way to us.

The next thing I knew, I was being taken to a room to monitor my son's heart. A kind doctor and knowledgeable midwife were requested and our thoughtful doula was called. Lots of rapid movements. Fast, fast, fast. They gave me gas but he was arriving quickly so it had little effect. I delivered with pure adrenaline. "Remember your breathing," my husband said. Our boy entered the world only two hours, eight minutes later at 7:08 am, weighing 6 pounds 12 ounces. It was insanely quick for a first baby because his heart rate dropped. I was in shock with him being three weeks early and with such an expeditious, intense delivery. It was an incredibly scary but phenomenal experience; my body powered forth my springtime baby into the world with an invigorating surge, so that his heart could beat strongly again.

I was amazed to meet him. His little face reminded me of a chestnut emerging from its shell or my hands after soaking in a warm, comforting bath. He soaked in and absorbed the warm comfort of my body. As I reached for him, he wriggled on my stomach and nuzzled his scrunched-up little face into my chest. I felt him latch straight away, and we were one again.

The day before I gave birth, we had my virtual baby shower. Some restrictions were lifted, so my parents and three close friends traveled to London and attended in person, with everyone else broadcast via video call on the large TV screen. My sister-in-law was convinced seeing my family and friends again and the flow of oxytocin, the happiness hormone, is what brought on my son's delivery three weeks early. I guess we'll never know, but it was a really special time and a wonderful introduction to life for my little boy.

Amazingly, his grandparents experienced my pregnancy for the first time and met their baby grandson, all in one weekend. There was something wonderful in hearing your parents tell you, "You're a complete natural." It was reassuring to know that even in the times I doubted whether I would be a good mum, they always knew I would be.

Every time people meet my son, the phrase I repeatedly hear is, "He is such a happy baby." Please don't mistake me; he cries when he needs something, but I also think my initial tough pregnancy experience made me pour my everything into him. Or perhaps this was the type of mother I was always destined to be—we will never know. I believe my commitment to him helps him be the joyous little boy he is.

I say my son saved me from my thoughts, but overall he saved me in a much greater way. He saved me from thinking that I wasn't worthy of being a mum. He saved me from living an unfulfilled life when I could be his mum and help others by sharing my story. I'm proud, and I'm grateful to be a strong mother, his mother.

THE TOOL

GET MOVING

This tool is extremely simple but effective. Get moving and reconnect with the world. Cycling in nature was such a phenomenal change for me. It's not just about pumping your body full of rich endorphins; it's about incorporating mindfulness, taking in your surroundings, and focusing on your breath.

Make it easy: James Clear mentions in his book *Atomic Habits*, "Reduce friction. Decrease the number of steps between you and your good habits." Make sure your cycling gear, kickboxing gloves, swimsuit, running leggings, or whatever sport it may be, is by your bedside or by the front door, ready to go!

Morning is best: Do your activity as early as possible. It's best to start your day with this before all else.

Nature is key: Exercising outside makes *all* the difference. Tune into the breeze on your skin as you take that badminton serve, feel the bumps in the road on your bike, watch the squirrels climb up the trees on your walk. Look at the rose, ocean blue or dark tempest of the sky, the seasonal hues of the leaves, feel the weather on your skin, take in the smells and sounds. You can live in the middle of the forest or a capital city, like me, and still find nature and connection.

Conscious breath: Be mindful and aware of your breath. This can be during the exercise or during a short break. Use the top three things you're grateful for on this particular day. Breathe these things in. Breathe in "I am grateful for brilliant career opportunities available for me to apply to." Breathe this in for four breaths.

Breathe out something negative in your life that you're not available for. "I am not available for gossip." Breathe this out for six.

Be conscious of your breath throughout your exercise.

You are living. Feel alive.

REFRAME YOUR THOUGHTS

You may have tried many gratitude processes, but the difference is that it goes in tandem with the first tool I mentioned (Get Moving).

Make it easy: Place a journal and a pen conveniently by your bed before you go to sleep.

When to do it: As you wake, write at least three things you're grateful for before exercising. You'll need to remember the top gratitude. If you can remember all three, even better.

What to write: Try to write something different every morning. Consider what happened the day before and what you're grateful for from that day. This will help you write something new.

If you're experiencing a difficult situation, look at what you're thankful for in that situation. "I am having a difficult relationship with someone," becomes "I am grateful for the help they've offered me over the years and the wonderful memories we share such as. . ."

What a fantastic way to start your day and a great way to reframe your worries.

Get moving. Get grateful. Two simple changes that changed and empowered me.

Often what feels like the terrifying, earth shattering, end is actually the most fantastic gift of a beautiful, crucial and euphoric beginning.

~Christina Morris

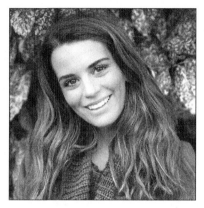

Christina is the owner of Yes Mama Mindset, where she coaches expectant mothers and helps them with self-belief and positive prioritization. She is the co-author of Black Belt Women and Lessons on Perseverance. She is a kickboxing black belt and Sensei. She loves yoga, pilates, swimming, martial arts with her son (the youngest in her dojo), solo cycling, and weightlifting. Christina loves to try new things and go to new places. She is also a Product Lead for an FTSE 100 tech company. She lives with her husband and son in London.

Website: yes-mindset.com

Facebook: facebook.com/yesmamamindset

Facebook profile: facebook.com/christina.morris.eleven

Instagram: Instagram.com/yesmamamindset

CHAPTER 2

THE MINDSET OF A STRONG MOTHER

THOUGHT MASTERY FOR HEALING AND MANIFESTATION

Laura Di Franco, MPT, Publisher

After almost thirty years of living 3000 miles away from my mom (who is 75 years old), I'm typing this on the afternoon she's due to arrive here in Maryland to start a new chapter of her life, five miles away from me! Mom hasn't lived anywhere but Northern California her entire life. My mom is a brave badass.

The feels: There's a little nugget of a knot in my throat. I'm proud of my mom.

After 53 years, I recently traveled out of the country by myself for the first time. I'm typing this chapter three days after returning from a shamanic healing writers retreat in Teotihuacan, Mexico, where I taught, and more importantly, received, for seven days. On the morning of my return, sitting down at Gate 52 in Mexico City, a young girl approaches me. "Would you please watch my backpack?"

Wait, didn't I just hear an announcement over the PA system warning us to call the airport police if anyone should approach us asking to watch their stuff? I felt the knowing prickle of hairs on the back of my neck.

"I can't watch your stuff, hun."

She walked away and didn't bother me again.

What, do I have a target on my forehead or something? Why me? "They look for certain kinds of people, Mom." My wise daughter. *What kind of person is that?*

I am also a brave badass. And I used to have to prove myself by making achievement and success a regular thing, by doing things I'd never done, just to say I did them. But after this trip, I made a decision. I don't want to travel by myself again. I just want to have more fun. I have nothing left to prove. I want to share all the magical moments with someone I love.

The feels: The ease and warmth around my heart settle in as I come to that conclusion. I hear you, soul.

After waiting over two years to face her abuser, my daughter will step into court this year because not telling was not an option. She'll change the lives of countless other young women with her courage. My daughter is a brave badass. And she'll be a strong mother one day.

The feels: It's the same throat knot this time. Tears well up with it. I can't hold them in. This is hard to choke down.

It's like a tiny me walking around. The desperate efforts to protect her are futile. Not being hurt by life is not an option for a strong mother, her daughter, or her mother or grandmother. It's the pain that we turn to passion and purpose, eventually.

Mom's mom died young from esophageal and breast cancer. They didn't have cigarette awareness when she grew up. Gram didn't have a chance to do a lot but survive. According to my mom, Gram was a brave badass.

Dad's mom died from non-Hodgkin's lymphoma. She spent her entire life catering to my grandpa, her four children (two of which she survived), and us grandchildren. I saw her light up when they spoke about travel. And that one time at my Gram and Gramp's 50th wedding anniversary—that was the biggest smile I ever saw on her face. She danced in Gramp's arms in the middle of the community center floor, and we all watched and clapped.

Why didn't we have more parties? She would have liked more parties, I'm sure of it.

The feels: Regret sits in the pit of my stomach, heavy and slightly nauseating.

Regret and guilt are pretty useless. I've learned to flip the switch when they show up. Mainly, I have to remember to honor any sadness. Then I must remember who and where I am now because this moment is the one worth living in—the only one worth my time, energy, and effort.

I've watched the women and mothers I love make decisions and live their lives based on fear or obligation. And I've watched some brave enough to choose their deepest desires. The year I chose joy over everything else was the most excruciating of my life. It meant another level of mindset training. It meant practicing awareness as a discipline and prioritizing myself. "I want a divorce." Those four words shattered everything. For the first time, I put myself in line in front of everyone else.

But you have kids. You're not allowed to put yourself first. Your job is to take care of them, make sure they have great lives. This might wreck them. What if this wrecks them?

"Be mindful of the needs of others." That was Mom's dad. That was passed down, for better or for worse, through the generations. Realizing that none of this is about me saved me many days. Helping others is purpose. Purpose will keep you from suffocating in the dark alley of your mind. But on other days, that phrase echoed in my head, accompanied by massive amounts of guilt. Remember what I said about guilt? Useless. Destructive. It's a soul-killer.

Many of us were taught we should come last. But the only true way to have the most amazing life, filled with enough energy, time, money, and resources to generously take care of ourselves and everyone we love, comes from prioritizing ourselves and our joy. That's a big-ass dilemma for many of us. We were never taught how to do it. Our models did the opposite in many cases.

The feels: There's a tightness somewhere between my chest and belly. It feels constricting and suffocating. I palm the center of my chest, hoping to rub it out. It's uncomfortable. It's been getting more intense lately.

"You better smell the smoke before your house burns down." The wise words of one of my coaches. She was talking about my marriage. I felt daily sharp pangs of chest pain.

You're going to die of a heart attack, and then what do you think will happen to the kids?

The inner voice had to start its campaign of tough love. She had to start teaching me what a truly strong mother meant. And that wasn't about ignoring my needs, desires, wants, or dreams anymore. It was about unapologetically going for the best possible life, the one I knew I was born for.

The feels: This crazy-ass smile widens across my face, and I can feel the sides of my mouth stretching. My chest and shoulders open up. My heart feels free. I sit taller on the bar stool. I feel solid. Unshakable.

Some of my bravest moments have been about learning the language of my soul and taking the risk to follow those messages. A strong mother can use vulnerability as strength and mistakes and failures as learning, growth, and opportunity. She can learn to discipline her mind in a way that she's always vibrating higher and emitting the energy of love and gratitude, no matter what is happening around her. Some days I think a strong mother is just someone who's not afraid to show you she's human and is willing to celebrate that, not taking a moment of this precious life for granted.

In Chapter 17, my friend Laura talked about the Warrior Mama. I love that! We are all warriors on this journey, showing up for the stuff of our lives and willing to fight the good fight for ourselves and those we love. We know what we're meant to do, what we were born for. We know we're worthy, even if it took a lifetime to get to that conclusion and do something about it. We are all actively healing the wounds, searching for joy, and living our moments by giving ourselves permission to feel everything—brave, badass warriors, indeed.

The mindset mastery started for me when I was taught to understand my body's language. The clarity and answers were there for me all along! Mindfulness is actually partly a practice of body awareness. Once I realized that feeling my way through life was the answer to many of the moments I had questions about, I stopped trying to analyze, problem-solve, and over-think my way through. All I had to do was pause, feel, notice, and then choose. With awareness—specifically body awareness first—I always had a choice. I moved from body awareness to thought awareness to mindset mastery.

I consider mindset mastery a lifelong practice, but one day I knew I'd arrived. I found myself deep in the pit of pain and despair, felt the tightness in my throat and chest, stopped the cyclical, ruminating negativity and worst-case thinking, and chose something healthier to think, believe, do, and say.

I can choose that path at any moment. It's the ultimate freedom. I get to create my life every moment, no matter what. As long as I stay awake and can feel and speak the language of my soul, I get to heal. And I get to set the stage for manifesting everything I desire. With this practice, you have to be careful what you wish for because you're likely to get it!

Let's start feeling together. Feeling is healing. Feeling is the gateway to all the answers you ever need in any moment of your life.

THE TOOL

When I began to understand the language of my soul and the messages being given to me daily in the form of sensations, feelings, and knowing, everything in my life changed. I realized thought mastery was more about feeling mastery. And I was no longer confused.

I now have badass clarity about my life and everything happening in it and never have to second-guess my decisions, even when other people tell me mine aren't right. I know for sure that they can't feel what I feel. Only I can feel what I feel and know if something is good or right for me. And that means I get to make choices based on that awareness. And so do you.

I want this kind of clarity for you. This exercise will help you connect with your intuition and internal GPS. It's about understanding how to feel your way through your life versus trying to think your way through when you're feeling confused, unclear, or unable to make a decision.

IS IT A HELL YES!? OR IS IT A HELL NO!?

What you need: A sheet of notebook paper and a pen.

Draw a line down the center of a piece of paper, so you have two columns. Label the top of the left-hand column "Hell No!" And label the top of the right-hand column "Hell Yes!"

Now, think about when something does not feel good to you. What does that feel like when a circumstance is a "no" for you? For example, when something isn't right or doesn't feel good to me, I feel tightness in my throat, and my body feels cold. I also feel weak, and my posture is slouched. My body tells me it's a "no."

In the left-hand column, under the label, "Hell No!" describe how that feels in your body for you. Make a list of words or descriptions for when something isn't right or doesn't feel good. See if you can come up with at least ten descriptive words or phrases and list them in that column.

Next, do the same for the right-hand column and the "Hell Yes!" Make a list of words or phrases that describe when things are amazing, feeling good, and you're feeling like everything is going your way. For example, when things are right for me, I feel light, strong, and warm, and there is a smile on my face. My posture is always tall and strong.

See if you can list at least ten words or phrases in the right-hand column for the "Hell Yes!"

Here are some of mine. Feel free to use them for your chart!

Hell No!	**Hell Yes!**
Tight	Light
Weak	Strong
Slouched posture	Open, tall posture
Cold	Warm
Frown	Smile
Foggy or unclear	Ease/clarity

What you've created here is a cheat sheet for your soul's language. Read your list. Every moment is an opportunity to feel what to lean into and what to walk away from. With awareness like this, you have a choice to make every good decision based on what will nourish you. What have you been saying yes to that was clearly a no? It's time to connect with your inner wisdom and choose what your soul is calling you to.

Now, think about when you're in a situation that feels confusing. You can't choose between the "Hell Yes!" and "Hell No!" What side does that go on? What is the feeling in that moment of uncertainty, fogginess, confusion, or lack of clarity?

I sat with one of my healers one day and stared out the beautiful top-floor window of her office at the trees. I was confused about my life and how I would take the risk and ask for a divorce. "It's easier to be confused," she said. "Then you don't have to make a decision."

In that one response, she woke me up to the fact that my confusion was certainly not a "Hell Yes!" My confusion felt nothing like when things were great, easy, and good for me. My confusion was the "Hell No!" It was clear. I was allowing myself to stay stuck there because I was afraid. This was a "no" message. I had a very difficult decision to make, and it would create freedom in my life like never before. The problem was that I was second-guessing the feeling and calling it "confusion" when it was a "no."

If you take responsibility for everything in your life, you'll see that life becomes a playground. The fear and uncertainty are there for you to develop your practice and mastery. It's an opportunity to understand yourself and your deepest desires. Discerning the real fear and "Hell No" from the purpose-driven fear is how you'll follow your heart and manifest everything you desire for your life.

IS IT FEAR OR PURPOSE-DRIVEN FEAR?

Part of mindset mastery is knowing the difference between those "Hell No!" moments and a feeling of purpose-driven fear. The problem is that they can feel very similar. However, the purpose-driven fear has a few characteristics that you can begin to notice so that when it shows up, you'll have an even more powerful cheat sheet for that soul language.

Here are the characteristics of those feelings:

Fear	Purpose-Driven Fear
Feelings of anxiety	Anxiety is overpowered by excitement
Not aligned with desires	Associated with something very aligned with desires
No bigger feeling	Sense of something bigger behind it
Random timing	Shows up over and over, like it wants your attention
Feels bad	Feels bad with a touch of excitement

What if, at any given moment, you had the secret code to making decisions that serve you and your greatest desires and purpose? These exercises are exactly that! Remember this is a daily practice, that when you master it, will help you access healing and manifestation at a whole other level.

After mastering body awareness and understanding the messages coming to you every day, you'll want to take your mastery practice to the next level and conquer the thinking mind. As you master your mindset and manifestation skills, you'll begin to live in awe of just what's possible for your life!

And Momma reader, you deserve the best, juiciest, most magical, magnificent life! When you live in the overflow, you get to generously take care of yourself and everyone you love. May that be the energy you move forward with each and every day from here on out!

The alarm bell now blares annoyingly from my iPhone.

It's time to go pick up my mom from the airport. I'm nervous and excited.

I'm blessed with knowing her last chapter will be with me, near me, and for me. I can't believe it's happening!

Mom, you are a brave badass. You are so amazing. I love you so much. I'm so grateful you made this big, bold, brave decision. I can't wait to have a chance to get to know you better, to sit for coffee, to cry, feel, and enjoy the pleasure of each other's company. I feel our healing moving across the generations to the Grams and Gramps, to my children, your grandchildren, and most definitely right here in the middle of my heart, which is a lot bigger because you are my mom.

I've missed you.

The feels: My heart explodes into a thousand pieces and heat, warmth, and light spread out from the center of my chest to my toes and fingertips. The tears come. Happy tears.

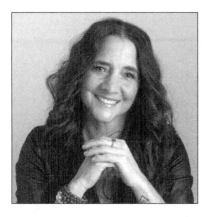

Laura Di Franco, MPT, is the CEO of Brave Healer Productions, specializing in publishing and business strategy for healers. She spent 30 years in holistic physical therapy and 12 of those in private practice before pivoting to publishing. With 14-years of training in the martial arts and 25 books and counting, including 27 Amazon bestsellers, she's got a preference for badass in every way.

Her daily mission is to help fellow wellness practitioners do what they need to do to change the world in less time and with fewer mistakes and heartache on the journey. She shares her authentic journey, wisdom, and expertise with refreshing transparency and straightforward badassery. Hold on to your seat because riding alongside her means you'll be pushed into and beyond your comfort zone and have way more fun with your purpose-driven fears on a regular basis.

When Laura chills out, you'll find her with a mojito at a poetry event with friends, driving her Mustang, bouncing to the beat at a rave, or on a beach in Mexico with something made of dark chocolate in her mouth.

Connect with Laura:

Website: BraveHealer.com

Facebook: https://www.facebook.com/BraveHealerbyLaura

Free Facebook Group:
https://www.facebook.com/groups/YourHighVibeBusiness

Instagram: https://Instagram.com/BraveHealerbyLaura

Twitter: https://Twitter.com/Brave_Healer

LinkedIn: https://www.linkedin.com/in/laura-di-franco-mpt-1b037a5/

YouTube:
https://www.youtube.com/channel/UCy5Ym97EetHuxpgJEHewwCQ

CHAPTER 3

I CAME LATE,
BUT I'M HERE NOW

CREATING PEACE IN THREE BREATHS

Atlantis Wolf

"[A] mother is one to whom you hurry when you are troubled."

-Emily Dickinson

MY STORY

I stood outside with chill bumps, numb toes, and a drippy nose beside my backed-in car, as the cold April rain-fed spring flowers still hibernated in the dark, wet ground, not ready to bring their nectar to the forthcoming summer sun. With the hatch open and halfway up the twin's driveway, I debated about waiting in the driver's seat. *No, they need to see me here, standing right outside the front door.*

"Get your shit outta here!" said the voice inside the house.

Jim came out first. "I'm carrying as much as I can, Mom," he said over his shoulder, carrying two boxes of sketchbooks and his cactus sprout collection balancing on top.

Grace, his twin, was half a step behind him. "I've got a bag of your clothes and a pair of shoes," she said to the back of his head, covered with his sweatshirt hood to protect against the steady rain.

I took each armful and organized it into the back. "Remember," I said, looking at them with steady, quiet eyes, "We're taking one load of Jim's stuff to my house, then we'll come back to get your stuff, Grace. If we need to make a third trip, we will. It's okay. Oh, ask for your birth certificates and social security cards."

"Here's more of your boxes," boomed the voice walking to the door. "See, I'm helping. I'm helping!" She looked at me from behind the screen door, pointing her finger, "And don't come in my house. You can't come in my house. It's my house!"

We were six feet apart. I forgot she had cut her long, ash-blonde hair to a pixie cut and dyed it the color of straw to see if her boyfriend loved her or her hair. I rarely saw her in person, just her kids, the twins. She was small and slender, like a fairy, so it was a constant surprise to hear her voice, aggressive and driving, like a bullet out of a gun—the crack of flint and the bang of startling sound.

"I'm staying right here, Becca," I said, anger warming my body as I watched her face, rain dripping off the end of the arm-sleeves of my winter coat, fingers folding closed.

Jim didn't have much, a favorite pair of vintage, high-waisted acid wash jeans, a collection of Japanese hooded sweatshirts, 80s nylon jackets, anime t-shirts, a pair of sneakers, old sketchbooks, favorite pencils, and a suitcase.

Grace sat on Jim's lap in the passenger seat next to me on the three-minute drive over the Rapid train tracks to my house.

"Mom's wonky today," Grace said.

"I know," I said. "We're going to come right back and get your stuff as fast as we can. It's okay."

"She said she's going to throw the cats outside because we're not there to take care of them," Grace said with tears in her widening eyes and emotion tightening her voice. "They're indoor cats."

"I didn't sign up for two extra cats, guys," I said, "But we'll work it out. It's okay."

We dropped the boxes at my house and grabbed two cat carriers from my basement.

Becca was waiting behind the screen door with her phone turned sideways. "See, Mom!" she said in a shrill voice, "There they go! Abandoning me! Look. Look!"

Jim and Grace walked past her with low shoulders, avoiding eye contact with their grandmother on video chat.

She's such a fucking nightmare, I thought to myself. *How does anyone survive that as your parent? I guess they had to come in as twins.*

I stood and waited, car running, breathing in the icy air and exhaling curls of steaming vapor from my nostrils. Across the road, through the veil of mist and rain droplets, I gazed at an empty lot, a rise of grass between two brick houses. I felt the sense of looking at something my eyes couldn't see. I looked back to the open front door.

As I waited, I remembered standing in the same place in the driveway with my car backed up the same way seven days ago, on a sunny afternoon with my kids, Andrew and Sofie, and four City Heights police officers, just after the twin's 18th birthday.

It was a plan seeded seven years ago when my daughter, Sophie, was telling a joke at her lunch table in fifth grade, laughing so hard her back bumped Grace's back behind her. "Hey, sorry, there," she said with her signature super-smile. "I'm Sophie." Sophie brought her into her friend circle that instant, and Jim a week later when they realized they were in the same cello class for band.

I knew the twins were strange and quiet, but so was I. It's okay. I struggled to plan playdates, movies, and dinners because they always had to ask their mom who wanted them to watch their half-brother, Dylan, eight years younger, while she and her boyfriend, Luke, worked. Even on weekends, there was always an excuse not to get together. They had to clean the house, do laundry, and work on homework. Eventually, I had them walk to my house on the way to high school so we could all have breakfast together and stay in touch. Waffles in the shape of the Death Star were a favorite. And always a pot of tea.

When the stories moved from Becca's binge-drinking to the twins having to bang on their ceiling at 3 am when Becca was having lusty make-up sex with her new boyfriend after their night-long fisticuff and flying objects fight, I knew an inevitable statement was coming. My first daughter, Sophie, looked at me from the breakfast table one morning and said, "Mom, we have to do something. We have to adopt them."

I'm a single mom with two kids and four cats, but I knew she was right. They just needed a chance, a safe place to try and stand up in the world. We all do.

Becca was a viper, a vicious alcoholic who once beat her boyfriend with his electric guitar while he was sleeping because she thought he was texting another woman. He wasn't. But she was having an affair with her art professor, so they broke up. My greatest fear was that she would beat the twins if they tried to leave.

Covid was not kind to kids who needed school lunches, teacher intervention, and peer interaction. We didn't see Jim or Grace for almost a year. Their mom kept them at home.

On their 17th birthday, we managed to take them out for a belated birthday dinner at their favorite Asian restaurant, where we sat on tatami mats, sipped tea, ate edamame, miso soup, and sushi. I held their hand, one each, across the table and said, "After your next birthday, I'm moving you out of your mom's house. You only have to make it for one more year." They looked at me with small shoulders and full bellies—a spark of hope.

A year later, I stood in their mom's driveway with my kids, Andrew and Sophie. We were instructed by the police to text the twins, back up the driveway, and wait for them to come outside.

Jim came out first, tripping with excitement, carrying his suitcase and Google Chromebook. "Mom's asleep!" he said.

"What?" I said with gathered eyebrows, "It's 2:30."

He put his two items in the back and got into the back seat. "She had a bad night and called in sick to work. She's right behind the door on the stuffed chair."

Grace followed right behind Jim, wearing the winter coat I gave her for Christmas. "I've got my suitcase and Chromebook," she said, "but I forgot my new sketchbook. Can I go get it?"

I looked at Officer Fuerst, his black uniform bulging over his flak jacket and belted arsenal of protection. "They can only take what is really theirs," he said.

I looked at the twins, knowing their sketchbooks were the most important possessions they owned. "Okay, both of you, go grab your sketchbooks but make it snappy. If your mom wakes up, just run back to the car."

They ran up the two steps and through the front door. *Slam!* The wood screen door smacked against the door frame, and the three of us jumped.

Their mom was legendary for how much she could drink, how many men she could bring home, and how ruthless she was in arguments. She would bob and weave like a cobra, twisting your words until you felt like you were arguing with yourself while recording the conversation on her phone to play back to you later—a real peach.

Slam! The twins came out with a handful of sketchbooks.

Slam! They went back in for their portfolio holders.

Slam! They came out with the portfolios and a box of brush pens.

Slam! They went back for paint, brushes, and trays.

Slam! They had enough to leave.

"Do we have to wake her up?" I said to Officer Fuerst, looking up into his blue eyes.

"No," he said. "I'm writing an incident report. I have your name, their names, her name, the address, and all the details. You just have to contact her, saying they moved out. That way, she can't report them as runaways."

"Can we text her?" I asked.

"Yes," he said.

We went home, unloaded the car, and texted her. We said we were in a hotel to keep her from coming to the house in a rage and tearing up my block. Not for the first time. I took the twins to my dad's house in the country and left them there with Sofie, prioritizing their physical safety for that first night. Andrew and I stayed at our house.

There was no incident. Eight years of holding our collective breath for the bomb that dropped. A dud. Their mom texted the next day that they could pick up their things Thursday.

And so I stand here on Thursday, one giant rip of the fabric of Becca's family as I wait to sew them onto the blanket of my family.

The door swings open. Grace says, "Mom is going to throw the cats out for real and isn't kidding and told Grandma, and we have to take them!"

"Okay," I say. "Put them in the carriers. Grab their food and litter box. They'll need familiar smells and familiar food."

Grace and Jim loaded a keyboard and stand, boxes of books and stuffed animals, bags of clothes, a bag of boots, a red cloak I gave her, a sewing machine, the down comforter and fleece blanket I gave her, two boxes of sketchbooks, a set of pots and pans from their grandmother, a mixer, mixing bowls, baking utensils, two cats, food, a litter box and a bag of stuffed animals. By the end, my car was stuffed, and they were squeezed into the passenger seat next to me, holding boxes labeled Time Capsule 1, 2, 3, etc., on Grace's lap.

"Is there anything else you need that's in the house?" I asked them. "Anything."

Their mom walked outside barefoot, stumbling down the wet steps and over to their side of the car. I rolled down the window halfway.

"And take this, Janice," she said, pushing the envelope at him. "It's your bill from the hospital. I made sure to put it in your name."

"It's Jim, Mom," he said.

"Well, I named you Janice," she said, weave-walking back to the house.

"This is your bill from the suicide night, isn't it?" I said, taking the envelope.

Jim nodded.

I ripped it into four pieces. "You were under 18 when it happened. You aren't liable; she is." I said. "And I have a date with the magistrate downtown. We're legally changing your name to James. It's okay."

Jim started to cry; Grace looked at him, her arm around his shoulders.

"No matter what happens to you for the rest of your life," I said, "It will be easier than that," pointing a thumb back at their mom's house. "Let's get some dinner."

We worked through each day talking and spending time together. It was 24/7 therapy. Over the first eight months, we traveled to Chicago for the twin's first trip to a big city (a delayed 18th birthday celebration), to Vermont to meet Grace's secret boyfriend, who she met in an online gaming community, and to the Caribbean to spend two weeks in each other's wounds, triggers, and fears until we came through as a family. It's ongoing.

A few weeks after they moved out, I took them to see their step-dad, Luke, and their half-brother, Dylan. It was always an easy relationship between the four of them, but they hadn't seen him in almost two years since their mom attacked him with his guitar while he slept.

I sat on the couch of Luke's ground floor duplex, watching him teach Jim how to strum a chord on his acoustic guitar while Dylan and Grace played with foam swords, making slow-motion dramatic gestures and sound effects. Grace was singing the song Luke was teaching Jim as it played on the record player. I sat content and smiling, at peace with the scene.

My eyes softened, and my clairvoyance reached out to feel another dimension to what I saw with my eyes. I saw spirit figures around the room in a circle, laughing and clapping at the scene. They were old women, ancient beings. They looked familiar. I wondered if these were the ancestors of the twins, their step-dad, and half-brother. But as one looked at me, I realized these were my ancestors, too. These women were common ancestors to the five of us from lifetimes ago, rejoicing at the reunion of family members, who orchestrated events to help us find each other.

I think of those women working behind the scenes when I tease Grace that she gets her bad eyesight and dyslexia from me. She does. It's just farther back than she realizes. And when I bought Jim a sports bra, swim trunks, and a sun shirt, so he didn't have to get his binder and t-shirt and shorts wet on vacation. His soul contract includes being transgender. Our common ancestors are wiping their brows and giving each other high fives that we all found each other again. And really, we are all family, all relatives.

EPILOGUE

Two-spirit figures, a man and woman, stand on a rise of grass, an empty lot between two brick houses in an inner-ring suburb, with their arms over the shoulders of three smaller figures. The cold April rain is falling, but they can't feel it.

"There she is," says the man. "That's her next to the car, standing in the rain."

"She's looking at us," says the smallest figure.

"She senses us," says the woman, "but she can't see us."

"Why did she get you?" says the smallest one.

"Because she's our mom," says the man, watching me. "It's what moms do."

THE TOOL

When new mothers ask me what kids are like, meaning babies, infants, tweens, and teens, I always answer with one word: relentless. Kids in all their forms are the embodiment of the life force, a continuum of needs, wants, changing appetites, and situations. My parenting goal is to launch sub-adults into the world with enough confidence to blossom into their full capacity. When they're excited about a new idea, I blow wind into their sails, and I make them popcorn and cocoa when things get weepy and bumpy.

What's the secret? For me, it's circular breathing. In three breaths, I can regain my ground and choose the next step. When the walls are crashing, I push the mental pause button, leave the scene (go to the bathroom, take my purse to my bedroom, walk around the aisle at the grocery store, etc.), and take three breaths. It never fails.

Circular breathing means in through your nose, slight pause, then out through your mouth as long and slow as you can manage. Think emptying the emotion of the moment from your toes up to your nose and another slight pause. Doing this three times resets your sympathetic nervous system, the fight-flight-freeze system, and allows you to balance the chemicals released into your kidneys from your adrenal glands. Your lungs are powerful detoxifying agents. Employ them.

Breath One: Close your eyes and breathe in a favorite place, like the beach, a wooded trail, or anywhere in nature. Imagine all the elements of nature coming to you to help. Pause. Breathe out and pretend you're emptying your lungs of every bit of air. Pause.

Breath Two: Keeping your eyes closed, breathe in more details of that place in nature, the sunshine on your face, the salt air in your nose, the smell of earth beneath your feet. Pause. Breathe out and pretend you are emptying your lungs and belly of every bit of tension. Pause.

Breath Three: Open your eyes and ground into your current environment. Breathe in this moment, knowing you're choosing how to react rather than being triggered by what is happening around you. Pause. Breathe out and imagine you're emptying your lungs, belly, legs, and toes of every last twinge of tension that was triggered in your body. Pause.

Ah, congratulations. You can now proceed in a place of grace and choosing. You are a beautiful mother, and your kids are the greatest investment of your time and attention. Thank you for volunteering to bring enlightened beings into the world. We need you.

I'm Atlantis Wolf, and I believe in you.

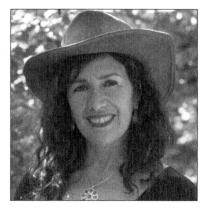

Emily Atlantis Wolf is a Shamanic Life Coach and workshop leader who helps people heal using licensed medical massage techniques, emotional release therapy, and spiritual guidance. Her joy is helping people discover their personal power by walking with them into their interior labyrinths, dark castles, and hidden stories. Her appointments are 90 minutes in-person or via Zoom and can be customized for any time zone in the world. She is a delight to invite to your podcast or public speaking event.

Atlantis grew up on a single-lane dirt road. She is sure her mother was an angel in human form as she whistled to birds and asked the question: "What am I being asked to do today?" Atlantis continues to walk into the forest at sunrise in all weather to ask that question every day.

She holds dual degrees in Civil Engineering and English with a minor in Environmental Engineering. Atlantis has worked as a civil engineer, technical writer, business analyst, project manager, licensed massage therapist, certified Emotion Code practitioner, marketing consultant, and entrepreneur.

She was spiritually asleep until events around her mother's death awakened her gifts to see and communicate with spiritual guides, power animals, and galactic dragons, remembering her past lives as an Egyptian healer, Toltec curandera, and Ayurvedic traveling shaman. She is the Dragon Medicine Woman.

Atlantis is an Aquarian, a single mom to four kids, three cats, and a hot cocoa connoisseur. She lives on Turtle Island.

Web: AtlantisWolf.com

Email: DragonMedicineWoman@gmail.com

YouTube: Atlantis Wolf

Instagram: @DragonMedicineWoman

CHAPTER 4

EVEN MOMS MAKE MISTAKES

WHY YOUR KIDS NEED TO SEE YOUR IMPERFECTIONS

Rev. Dr. Ahriana Platten

Every cell in my body screamed, *I'm not ready! I don't know how to be a mom yet!*

MY STORY

"Let's have that baby today," the obstetrician said with an authoritarian air. "I know you're not due for a couple of weeks, but the baby is plenty big enough, and there's no good reason to wait."

I have a good reason to wait! I don't know how to do this!

Tears filled my eyes, but he never noticed. I choked on my fear, and the words in my head couldn't seem to find their way out of my mouth. He called hospital admittance, and I was quickly seated in a wheelchair and shuttled across the hospital building by an intern. I didn't know until afterward that Dr. Rush-A-Lot wanted to go on vacation the next day. That was his *expert* reason for inducing labor.

At 19, I was too young to question his opinion. Being pregnant at that age wasn't in my playbook. I'd only been married six weeks when I conceived my son. In that short time, I had enough awful experiences to know I was married to an abuser. The next nine months were a blur of marital insanity. I won't go into it, but suffice it to say, I didn't have much time to think about becoming a mom.

When the doctor suggested inducing labor, I suddenly felt completely unprepared. Just weeks earlier, I was so tired of being pregnant that I was anxious to give birth. How hard could this mothering thing be, anyway? Hold them. Feed them. Change them. Love them. I thought I had all the tools I'd need to do those things. After all, I'd been babysitting since I was 12, and I helped my mom care for my three little brothers my whole life. That was enough preparation for motherhood, right?

What resulted from the doctor's haste was a horrible experience that involved breaking my water, an intravenous Pitocin drip that made me throw up repeatedly, 36 hours of torturous labor, and an eventual epidural to numb the unbearable pain. In the end, I tearfully held my beautiful baby boy in my arms—exhausted and broken. Within 24 hours of his birth, Josh's face was completely black and blue, and he was suffering from a birth-sustained broken collarbone that caused him to cry every time I held him. No one realized his collar bone was broken until his six-week check-up, so I assumed I was holding him wrong and, no matter what I tried, he cried every time he was in my arms for the first month and a half.

During labor, the medication I was given made my baby so sick that Josh's little tummy rejected the milk every time he ate. After the third time he vomited, the attending nurse said, "Don't worry, honey! You just rest. I'll take him to the nursery, and we'll take care of him for you." Once again, the objecting voice in my head was unable to utter a sound. Before I could speak, I was left alone, and my baby was whisked out the door in a flurry of scrubs and swaddling.

If I can't feed him or hold him without hurting him, what am I going to do when I get him home?

For several hours, all I could do was cry. I was a failure on the very first day of motherhood. I'd been so sure I could be a perfect mom without any additional preparation beyond the little childhood babysitting experience.

What's a perfect mom? You know, her children adore her. She's a complex mix of a nutritionist, playtime pal, home educator, seamstress, and life coach, all wrapped up in elegance and effervescent smile and equipped with perfectly timed intuition. When her child bellows its first breathtaking cry, a perfect mom is magically endowed with ancient mothering secrets that guide her every step on the parenting path. She knows when to be soft and when to be tough, what questions to ask at school conferences, and how to use tin foil, a magic marker, strips of fabric, and a few odd buttons to *McGyver* a one-of-a-kind Halloween costume. She finds more than enough time to balance nurturing her children with loving her partner and engaging in a satisfying and world-impacting career. This mythical creature can do it all—and she makes it look easy!

Did you catch that word? Mythical? Just like your fairy godmother. It took me the better part of forty years of mothering to realize the reason the perfect mother is best friends with Santa, the Easter Bunny, and the Tooth Fairy is that they all have one thing in common: they don't exist. And, despite the commercialized images gracing magazine covers and grocery store displays, perfect moms could never really give children what they need.

Why would anyone want to be perfect in the first place?

For me, it's always been because the opinions of my children mean more to me than the opinions of just about anyone else on the planet. I want to be the cool mom, the mom who always has the best snacks, the mom their friends wish they had! If I'm perfect, maybe they'll love me as much as I love them!

Children need us to make mistakes and show them how to offer a sincere apology. They need us to confront self-doubt and work through it so we can light the path for them when they face their own self-doubt. They need us to share our tears when a loved one dies, to be tired after a long day's work, and to forget things we meant to bring with us on vacation. They need us to fall, dust ourselves off, and get back up again, so they can learn how to handle their own failures. They're counting on us to demonstrate our imperfections so they can figure out how to deal with their own.

As I write this, I have five kids ranging in age from 19 to 41. I've been parenting longer than most people ever will, and I've been a grandma almost as long as my youngest son has been alive.

From stinky diapers to crayon-decorated walls, from middle school relationship drama to beer-can-strewn college parties, from losing a job they loved to the heart-wrenching experience of watching them leave home for a job in another country, I've shuffled my way through the challenges of motherhood in less than perfect ways and my children are better people for having seen my flaws.

You see, kids will make mistakes. It's how they learn. They'll throw temper tantrums, tell us they hate us, sneak out at night, and hide less-than-straight-A report cards. Important notes from teachers will disappear into the great abyss at the bottom of their backpacks, dogs will eat reams of undone homework, and little white lies will unlock certain freedoms sooner than we'd have granted them. That's all part of being a kid. And each child is different and has different needs. Just about the time you think you have this mothering thing mastered, one of your kids will pull a stunt you never anticipated. That's motherhood.

Being a mom is a lifetime commitment. Some of the biggest challenges of motherhood come after our children are grown when they face heartbreak, professional failures, and the bumps and bruises that come with facing their own parental flaws. If you've worked their whole life to be the perfect mom, how will they feel safe asking your advice when it comes to parenting your grandchildren?

Embrace your imperfections. Do it now. No matter where you are on your mothering journey, it's time to give up the myth of the perfect mom. Motherhood is all about learning, and kids are life's greatest teachers. Your job is to love your kids. Love is the first and most important gift you can give them. When you love them through their mistakes, they learn to love you through yours. They also learn that making a mistake doesn't make a person unlovable. Releasing the expectation of perfection allows them and you to be courageously, authentically, human.

To be clear, I'm not giving permission for anyone to subject kids to unhealthy addictions, abuse, or neglect. These are extremes that no child should endure. I'm talking about letting your kids see you as a human being who faces the day-to-day ups and downs of life. After all, they're going to explore those hills and valleys themselves at some point. When they learn about the challenges you've faced, they're more likely to believe you can relate to what they're going through.

Oh, you'll still hear, "You're too old to understand," "The world is different now," and, "I have to figure this out myself, Mom." If your children know you aren't perfect and have made your own mistakes, it will be easier for them to reach out to you in some of their hardest moments. Moments when they make big mistakes. Moments when they feel like they've failed. Moments when they don't like themselves very much. And those hard moments are when they really need you.

So, are you ready to be imperfect?

THE TOOL

To embrace your imperfections, you'll have to be willing to do a little soul-level work.

First, you'll need to be blissfully honest with yourself. If you make a mistake, admit it. Sit with the feelings you're having. Specifically, what's the mistake? And, how do you know you've made a mistake?

When I make a mistake, I often feel a knot in my throat or in my stomach. Something just doesn't feel right inside me. I begin by exploring the motivation for my actions. Often, I recognize that I'm operating from fear rather than love. More often than I care to admit—I'm trying to control my child because I'm afraid for them. Instead of talking through my concerns with them, I simply say 'no' or try to impose a better idea on them. I can't see it at the moment, but something tells me, after the fact, that I screwed up.

What's your inner mistake signal? What tells you to stop and reconsider? Learn what your signals are and pay attention to them. Consider your motivations. Ask yourself what outcome you're after and why that outcome is important to you. If you're being led by fear, work through it with a partner or a friend before you try to talk to your child about it. You may find that your fear has nothing to do with your child and a lot to do with your own life experiences. And, once you identify your mistake and understand why you made it, gift your child with a sincere apology.

Next, learn to laugh. Humans are funny. Making a mistake isn't very often the end of the world. It may be the beginning of a new way of being. Do your best to see the humor in being a mom. Here's an example:

Getting my youngest out of bed is challenging; he loves to sleep in. When he was young, our early morning dialogue often went something like this:

"Good morning, sweetheart. It's time to get up," I say softly.

Silence.

"Come on, son. You'll be late," I say a little louder.

Silence.

"HEY! I mean it! Get! Up!" I say much louder.

Without even opening his eyes, the seven-year-old responds: "The person you're trying to wake is not here right now. Please leave a message after the sleep. Sleeeeeeeeeep."

I busted out laughing! And I still laugh about it today! He didn't get up and was, indeed, late for school. We both laughed. I've replayed that scene in my head for years. Funny moments become treasured childhood memories, and they're way more important than being late for school on occasion.

Laugh often. Laugh out loud. Write the funny moments in your journal or share them on your social media and help other moms laugh. Every mom needs a good laugh! Laughing at mothering, in general, helps all of us to love the most uncomfortable and unexpected aspects of motherhood. If you're having trouble laughing at yourself, watch recordings of funny mom comediennes like Ali Wong, Anna Farris, or Kristin Hensley and Jen Smedley of *#IMomSoHard*. Christina Pazsitzky's *Mother Inferior* special is hilarious. Be warned, though it's a little off-color and not suitable for watching with the kids or with husbands whose sense of humor is lacking.

Step three, notice the compassion you give others and give it to yourself in the same measure. We can be so forgiving of other people's behaviors and eccentricities, can't we? If a guest in your home opens the refrigerator and the jelly jar falls off the shelf and comes crashing to the floor in a shattered mess of gooey glass shards, you'll most likely say something like, "Are you okay? Don't worry! It's just jelly. We'll clean it up." On the other hand, if you open the refrigerator door yourself and the jelly jar falls off the shelf and crashes to the floor, making a huge mess, it's likely the words that cross your mind are best expressed in a series of symbols! "Sh*t! What the h@*l! D@#mm*t! I don't have time for this!"

Befriending the inner critic and learning to speak to yourself with the compassion and the kindness you use to speak to other people is so important for you and for your kids. You deserve to be treated with the same love and respect you give to others. Be kind to yourself. Be gentle with the words you use to describe yourself. For most of us, it feels awkward to look in the mirror each day and say "I love you" to the reflection in your mirror, however, it's a life-changing exercise. Doing it might make you cry the first few times—do it anyway. And keep doing it. Look at your beautiful self for as long as you can and tell yourself what you love about yourself. Over time, you'll begin to believe yourself.

Finally, remember that kids are resilient. Give some thought to the number of crazy things you did as a kid. Instead of focusing on how dangerous or harmful those things seem to you now, think about how much fun you had, how you easily survived, even thrived despite your childhood adventures. Children are much more resilient than we give them credit for. Broken bones mend, and broken hearts open us to deeper understandings about life. Kids need to know they can recover when they make mistakes (*especially* when they make big mistakes). One of the hardest truths each of us must come to grips with is that we can make choices, but we can't choose the consequences of those choices. Every child will experience pain, no matter how hard we work to protect them. Pain is part of life, and it's foundational to wisdom. We can't protect them from experiencing pain in the long run, but if we're willing to show our flaws and faux pas, we can show them how to handle it.

"The only true sin is to steal your child's lessons," a respected elder once told me. That advice rings in my ears every time I find myself wanting to rescue one of my children from a tough situation. I know, I know—it hurts to see our kids hurt. The thing is, each of us, including our children, is here to live life. Our work is to guide our children, not stifle them.

In closing, let's consider the title of this book: *Strong Mothers*. The strongest mothers I know are real, raw, and honest. Being a strong mother requires a willingness to be truly seen, in your most vulnerable moments, by those you love the most. At some point, being seen will subject you to your children's judgment. Let me tell you a little secret about that; they're going to judge you no matter what you do. Every moment they're with you, they're watching and learning from you, judging whether what you say and do is right or wrong. It's how they grow and learn. Let them see the real you with all your imperfections. We're not here to be perfect; we're here to love each other, despite our imperfections.

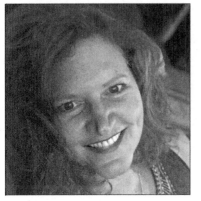

Rev. Dr. Ahriana Platten, Priestess, Pastor, Peacemaker. Ahriana is an international speaker, best-selling author, and courage builder who helps people find their sacred purpose and live from it. She's a master ceremonialist and practical mystic widely appreciated for her authenticity, professional insights, and coaching on the change process.

As the founder of Asoulfullworld.com, Ahriana leads a global wisdom community offering leading-edge spiritual teachings and tools for transformation. She describes her community this way:

"At Soul-Full, we provide a spiritual foundation not reliant upon dogmatic beliefs or creed yet honoring of an individual's religious devotion. We're sensitive to the seasons and cycles of nature and the ways living in harmony with the earth improves our lives. We value the arts – music, writing, dancing, painting, and more as spiritual experiences and tools for transcendence. We understand that the inner landscape is foundational to the discovery of a person's true nature, and we explore and cultivate peace and ease in the mind, body, heart, and soul. We equally understand that shaping the world is both our privilege and our responsibility, and we provide initiatives and education to support global healing and transformation."

She's the mother of five boys and has seven grandchildren and two great-grandchildren. She shares her life with her amazing husband, Mark, who loves her despite her imperfections.

Connect with Ahriana:
On her website: https://www.asoulfullworld.com
On Facebook: https://www.facebook.com/ahriana.platten/ or
https://www.facebook.com/groups/soulfully
On Instagram: https://www.instagram.com/ahriana_platten/

You'll find a free guided meditation and other gifts at
www.asoulfullworld.com

CHAPTER 5

BECOMING A STRONG MOM

THE BIRTH OF SELF ADVOCACY

Jacqueline M. Kane, R.T., LMT, EFT,
Bowen Therapy Practitioner

MY STORY

THE BIRTH OF SELF ADVOCACY

Ever since I can remember, I knew I was going to have children. It was something I always desired.

A few years into my marriage, I was excited to announce to my family and friends that I was pregnant. As much as I was looking forward to having them, nothing prepared me for the challenges I would experience with my children. Unfortunately, children don't come with directions or a how-to guide.

My husband and I were excited and a little scared. After all, this would be a first child for both of us. We were going to experience many firsts over the next 20 years. As much as I'm a planner, there was no planning for this.

My pregnancy with my first son was easy compared to what some women go through. There was no morning sickness or nausea. My only problem was that I loved food way too much and gave myself permission to eat as much as I wanted. My taste buds were on high alert. Everything tasted so yummy and satisfying that I just kept eating. My body didn't have that full feeling sensation. It was full steam ahead, and my body asked for more and more. I was not about to deprive it!

On my last appointment, my doctor casually stated, "Let's pick a day and time for your C-section," as if he was ordering his lunch. The ultrasound scan informed him that the baby was larger than most and that a cesarean operation was the best option.

Hours later, it felt like my entire world was crashing down on me. As I was cooking dinner and clutching the refrigerator door, I heard the words, "OMG, this is my worst nightmare. I don't want to have a C-section; that's not what I planned."

At the time, I worked in a hospital and saw what happens behind closed doors. I saw naked bodies on surgical tables, and didn't want that for me. I gained a ton of weight during my pregnancy and was embarrassed by how large I felt.

And I didn't want to be cut open. Even though I worked in a hospital, I didn't always agree with the care patients received. I have a deep sense of respect for doing things naturally, and a surgical procedure was not natural in my eyes.

I was disappointed, scared, and just freaking out about what my doctor decided was the best way to deliver my baby. My due date came and went, and my body was showing no signs of contractions or anything close to being ready to give birth.

Over a few days, there were numerous phone calls to friends and anyone who would listen to a nervous first-time pregnant woman looking for support and guidance. My mind was obsessed. *What if something goes wrong? What's recovery like from surgery? How will I be cared for?*

Surgery and being a patient were not what I planned. My pregnancy hormones were out of control, so were my emotions. My doctor decided, and it seemed I had no choice but to go along with it. I resigned myself and agreed.

I discovered a good side to having a C-section—scheduling. The doctor and I agreed on a date that made it easy for my husband to take time off work to be there for the special day. This was convenient compared to being surprised by the baby deciding, "Today's the day; think I'll show up now."

We arrived at the hospital. The nurse checking me in asked, "You're scheduled for a C-section, right?"

"Yes, even though it's not what I really want," I replied.

"Well, we could talk to the doctor about getting you induced. Is that something you want information about?" The nurses surprised me by listening to my fears about surgery and talking to me about options.

I felt hope rise inside of me as I said, "Yes, what would that involve?" They explained the procedure. "Yes, let's talk about that."

This was my first experience being a patient in a hospital, so there were lots of unknowns. I had to put my trust in someone else and pray they knew what was best for me.

My experience with doctors was that they thought they knew best and told me what would happen. The nurses shared a different option, then asked me what I wanted to do. *Why hadn't the doctor shared that option with me instead of planning to cut with a knife as the first choice?*

This was the first time in my life I felt I was being seen, heard, and listened to. The nurses and I formed a team, and the doctor agreed to a plan and joined in. He was not the only one making the decision for how this birth would go. I could be induced.

There were parts of this decision I loved and parts that were not so great. Being induced meant I would be allowed to eat nothing but ice chips. It meant I'd be hooked up to IVs, and machines with incessant bings, beeps, and alarms.

There was no permission to walk the hospital halls waiting for my water to break or anyone massaging my back. For the next hours, I'd be confined to a bed and hooked up to machines to monitor the health of the baby until my cervix was dilated enough for me to push.

The excitement of this entire ordeal was rubbing off as I watched one hour run into the next. I was getting bored lying in bed with nothing to do but wait, feeling uncomfortable, and thinking about the food I wasn't allowed to eat.

It was sweet to see my mother-in-law bring my husband a brown bag of food and watch him eat a wonderful sandwich she made with love for her son to make sure he was taken care of during his stressful time awaiting his first child. I was starving and would have loved just a bite, but I didn't say anything to him. "Go ahead, honey. You enjoy it."

Back then I was always the good girl, so I didn't want him to feel bad for eating food in front of a starving pregnant woman. That was when I didn't advocate for myself. So much has changed since that day. Now I speak up.

About 25 hours into the induction, my inner voice started talking to me. *Oh man, why did I not want a C-section? Now look at you: 25 hours and you are exhausted. You should have gone for the C-section.*

When I rolled over from lying on one side to the other, this would create a rush of five staff members asking, "What's going on?" Unbeknownst to me, the monitors would alarm every time I turned over, registering that something was wrong, even though there wasn't.

They checked on the baby and me every time. I finally learned to try and stay still as much as I could.

Finally, during the 26th hour of being on my back, there was a twinge. "I think I feel something?"

The nurse replied, "Great, let's see if you are dilating." She checked. "Yes, you are dilated, and it's time to push."

I felt relief, then. . . *You want me to push after not eating for over 26 hours?* My body was exhausted, and I just wanted it over. My sweet husband said, "Hey honey, this is what we wanted," but he wasn't the one lying on the bed.

"Really? That's easy for you to say after being fed and hanging out." As tired as I was, I knew he was right. After all, I was delivering my first baby the way I wanted—vaginally, not by C-section.

After a few good pushes, our first son Patrick Nicholas Kane came into the world. There are no words to express the love and joy that came with seeing my child for the very first time. For the first time in my life, I felt what true love is in my heart. My joy and unconditional love overflowed for this new human being that my husband and I created. There were no words to express the emotions. All of a sudden, it was all worth it. Patrick Nickolas Kane weighed 9 pounds, 11 ounces. The ultrasound was right; we had a large baby.

There were moments when the nurses would keep Patrick in the nursery so I could get some rest. We laughed as everyone compared him to the delicate smaller babies in the nursery. He looked like a three-month-old compared to them.

To me, he was a perfect size. He felt like a comfortable blanket as I held him on my chest and rocked him to sleep. He gave me the greatest gift of becoming a mom, and I was blessed to have him.

My life became all about him. When Patrick needed something, he cried to let me know it. As a first-time mom, I tried to be the perfect mom with the perfect baby. He was colicky a lot, and there were many times I had no idea what he needed. Some days were tough trying to figure out what he needed. Of course, many people shared their suggestions, saying, "Do it this way. And try this." Or, "Patrick needs this."

The good thing with babies is that they grow so fast that in a few months, one habit will go away, and another one will appear. My only regret was that I cared too much about having everything perfect and could have spent more time just letting the dishes pile up while I enjoyed having him in my arms as we sat in the rocking chair.

My days revolved around the clock and the next feeding. Breastfeeding was a little tricky for such a big, hungry boy. I was desperate to get him on real food, hoping it would fill him up and we could go longer between feedings. This gave me an opportunity to advocate for my son. I asked the doctor if we could start him on baby food earlier than normal. It seemed like he was always hungry.

Wouldn't it seem normal that a bigger baby can switch to regular food sooner than later? As an Italian mom, one of my greatest pleasures is cooking delicious meals for family and friends. It made me so happy seeing

Patrick's love for food. No wonder food was my simple pleasure while I was pregnant. This kid was going to love all kinds of food!

There were so many questions as a first-time mom. Of course, everyone was more than happy to give their suggestions and ideas of what my son needed or tell us how to take care of him.

There would be times when I enjoyed having help and recommendations, and then other times when I would have preferred to be asked, "Would you like some help? Are you all set?"

Asking someone if they are all set lets them know they are capable and instills trust and confidence. In my upbringing, there wasn't a lot of support. This translated into wanting to support my children to instill confidence and self-esteem, so I parented differently than how I was raised.

In order to become the parent I never had, I had to unlearn my conditioned patterns and learn a new way of being. It wasn't easy in the beginning, and there were many mistakes along the way. Thank goodness, with practice, I've been able to raise my kids in an environment where they feel comfortable being themselves. They have become confident, young caring men. I'm proud to be their mom.

Since giving birth to Patrick, I have shifted careers and am excited to say that I'm passionate about helping moms feel good and have all the energy they need to take care of their families.

As a master energetic healer, I now get to guide women to uncover their hidden energetic and karmic blocks that keep them in physical, emotional, and financial pain. By using my Get to the Root Cause process, we unravel negative thoughts and clear limitations, including Inner Child and Ancestral Karma, that hold them back, sometimes for decades. My clients are able to quickly and easily achieve major shifts creating a new level of health, wealth, and lifestyle that they desire now.

Here is one of my favorite tools to share with all of you amazing moms.

THE TOOL

Many moms are overwhelmed with a long to-do list, so I wanted to give you an easy tool to use.

If you enjoy listening to a meditation, you can go to my resource page and enjoy a guided meditation. I originally shared it in my co-authored book, *The Ancestors Within*, available on Amazon.com.

In this ten-minute guided meditation, I'll lead you on a journey to help you release energetic generational patterns that are stored in your body so you can reclaim your energy and activate your soul's authentic alignment. When used daily, you'll have a respite from the chatter in your mind, align with your soul's purpose and feel loved.

https://jacquelinemkane.com/resources/

I would love to hear what you thought of this meditation, so feel free to email me at jacqueline@jacquelinemkane.com.

My tool to share is for you to create *My Sacred Mom Time Out Daily Practice*, no matter how old your children are. Here are my guidelines and steps to creating what that could be for you.

STEP 1: AWARENESS

- Make a list of the five to ten habits that excite you and energize you, for example, taking a bath, reading, alone time, hiking, talking to a friend, etc.
- Set aside time daily to do one of those habits.
- Be committed to yourself and creating your sacred space.

STEP 2: ENERGY MAINTENANCE

- Make a habit of tuning in to your energy throughout the day so that you stay stress-free and create a safe environment for your children.
- Confident children are raised in an environment where they feel safe to ask for their needs and safe to express their emotions.

- Notice what you're feeling. Are you tired, stressed, or not present? Acknowledge when you're tired and give yourself permission to lay down and take a nap. If you're depleted, then everything you do will have that exhausted energy in it and it won't feel good, or you will get frustrated that it's not happening the way you desire. In those moments, walk away and give yourself a mommy time-out. You deserve it.

- By doing this, you'll show your children that it's okay to feel all of your emotions and feelings. It's safe to express the real you. You are your children's first teacher.

STEP 3: ENJOY YOURSELF

- When we feel joy in our hearts, people feel it. The more joy we feel in raising children, the more we will heal the world.

- Expand into joy every single day. Infuse your day with it. Create your joyful, passionate routine so you have all the energy you need to take care of yourself and your family. I promise you your life will be overflowing with ease, flow, and abundance, and your children will love you for it.

Being a mom is the greatest gift and can be the hardest job you will ever have. Be patient with yourself when things don't go well and know that everything is happening as it should. Take a breath and then another and celebrate what you have created and all you have accomplished. You are amazing.

Let's connect and share our stories.

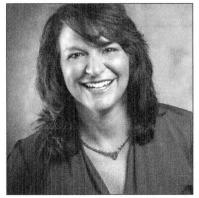

Jacqueline M. Kane is a Master Energetic Healer who guides women to uncover their hidden energetic and karmic blocks that keep them in physical, emotional, and financial pain. Using her Uncover The Root Cause process, we unravel negative thoughts and clear limitations, including Inner Child and Ancestral Karma, which has held them back for decades.

With over 20-years in private practice as a healer and over 35-years in health care, Jacqueline has merged her innate wisdom with a multitude of healing modalities, including Bowenwork, Emotional Freedom Technique, Evolutionary Meditation, Soul Clearing, and more to create unique, results-oriented methods for healing. Her clients are able to quickly and easily achieve major shifts to create a new level of health, wealth, and lifestyle they desire now.

Jacqueline's powerful programs, available to individuals, groups, and organizations, liberate clients from both physical pain and financial struggle, so they create a path to energy, health, the ease with money, and personal fulfillment. She is the creator of the *Healthy Wealthy Success System©* that guides women in creating a life filled with power, pleasure, and passion.

When Jacquelines' not working, she enjoys bike rides with my husband on their electric bikes, golfing with family and friends, and traveling to new exciting destinations.

You can connect with her:

On her website: www.JacquelineMKane.com

On Facebook: https://www.facebook.com/jacqueline.kane.313/

Facebook Group:

https://www.facebook.com/groups/healingcirclebyjacquelinekane/

On LinkedIn: https://www.linkedin.com/in/jacquelinekane/

CHAPTER 6

AM I ENOUGH?

THE ART OF LETTING GO

Layne Eliese Mills

MY STORY

I can feel the black hole in my stomach growing larger, consuming my self-confidence and replacing it with doubt.

You have to do this. I plead with myself. *You cannot keep pretending everything is okay. It's time to let it go.*

The voice is right. I hold my phone in one sweaty palm and press dial with the other hand.

"Hi, it's Layne,"

This is someone I consider a friend! Why am I so worried?

"So, I'm calling because, well, I'm sorry, but I'm not going be doing music lessons anymore." What I couldn't tell her at the time was how vibrant my internal life had become over the last year, speaking online with people all over the world about spirituality, and that teaching music lessons no longer felt *right* in my life. I was still too afraid to admit it.

"Oh! Okay." I can hear her disappointment. *If I'm not doing the lessons for her kids, is she still my friend?*

All of my students love coming to my house for their piano, ukulele, guitar, and singing lessons. Honestly, I loved seeing them and their excitement. Every win was my win because I had the privilege of showing them the secret of using their fingers just right to produce the sound they wanted from their instrument. I would visit with their moms while their siblings took turns playing with my kids. It felt so good to know I was actually using the degree I went to college for after all these years and having kids of my own.

Two years prior to that phone call, I felt that I'd barely begun to embody a version of motherhood that felt successful after being a stay-at-home mom for the last six years. I have two boys, the youngest about to start pre-kindergarten full-time without me, and the oldest in first grade. I now had an opportunity to work and make some money in a way that served my community. I thought this was it. It was good and was right for me. I thought I had finally arrived. Then, in the spring of 2019, I found out I was pregnant, again.

My baby was due in January 2020, so I decided to keep working all the way through to the end of 2019. When it was finally time for the Christmas program, I was so ready to be done at a full, humongous eight months pregnant. I said my goodbyes to all the families I worked with, and left it open on my end.

"I'll be in touch! I want to give myself plenty of time to heal and rest with my new baby before I start up lessons again." Everyone understood, and no one questioned it.

Knowing I was going to have some downtime with the baby, I also signed myself up for an online Master's Program in Elementary Education.

It will be good to go ahead and get my teacher's licensure since I'm actually teaching! I can do a couple of hours a day towards school with the baby hanging out, and his big brothers are off to school.

It'll be easy.

My famous last words. I had zero clue what was coming. To be fair, no one else did either.

This was the year of Covid. This was the year my oldest came home for spring break week, which then turned into two weeks, and then became indefinite. I was forced to choose homeschooling or distance learning.

It was a mess—a complete disaster. My kid was fighting with me while I tried to get him to listen to a short video and think about it thoroughly enough to answer a few questions. It was a joke how easy the material was, but he still fought me every step of the way. Everyone knows me as the teacher, and yet I hadn't changed out of my sweats and pajamas for months. I was constantly behind on my own homework, which was mindless work. Everything I wrote about with regard to teaching in the classroom was already so dated. Now I was looking ahead at our kids and their empty classrooms with plastic dividers wondering why I was writing lesson plans in college that include children working in small collaborative groups.

At the first sign of our school opening back up to students, we were there, but I felt like a failure. I couldn't even teach my own kid. I couldn't keep up enough in my own studies to pass my classes. I was at risk of losing my financial aid.

Like most people around this time, I turned to social media for a distraction. I happened upon some Facebook groups whose focus was on the exploration of spiritual matters. I hadn't encountered that before, and I became curious. *What was this?* Some of them felt so 'out there.' There was new-age, alchemy, esoteric occult, and even witchcraft.

That's interesting, I thought. *I wonder what they talk about in here?*

I was raised Catholic, and at five years old, informed that I was damned, that I was a bastard child of the church and condemned to Hell because of choices my parents made. Both were married before, and therefore their current marriage was not recognized by the church. I was shocked, disillusioned, and bereft. I looked up to Sister Kathleen and the Nunnery as a path to Spirit, and I was forced by this event to look elsewhere for closeness with the Creator.

From that moment on, I was in a state of constant spiritual curiosity, looking for answers. I couldn't believe that God imbued me with so much love, and so much wonder in my heart, and a burning hunger to know Him better, only to be told that, somehow, I was unworthy because of other people's choices. I was told that God Almighty had, without trial or comment, condemned me straight to Hell.

I've studied many disciplines and as many religious beliefs as I could with the time I had at my disposal. I felt I had as good a grip on what spirituality looked like with what I taught myself when I found the Facebook groups.

I realized these were just normal people trying to navigate the gray areas and the gaps in between various religious dogma. And I realized they were filled with questions that *I* had answers to! At best, they were all seeking the same things—the things I was working to understand. All of them striving to know what their place is in the world and how they not only fit in but how they can create the life they dream of.

All my little curious interests came together and culminated into this greater understanding. I was suddenly in a position to give advice and guidance on what I feel is the most interesting topic, the Spirit. Our Spirit. And our purpose here with it.

This is what I want to do.

But how? How do you go from doing work that everyone in your community respects to 'whatever this is'?

I decided I could figure out what *this was* later, but for the time being, I had to let go of a whole bunch of junk I'd been carrying around with me. The first and heaviest being my own internal expectations.

I built up all kinds of ideas about who I am. *Who am I supposed to be? What is that person supposed to look like in the eyes of my parents or my peers?* I thought I had to be the mom who had her act together—the teacher-mom, whose kids had killer high IQs because she knew just how to teach them, and everyone else's kids, too. I needed to be busy, busy, busy! I thought I needed to hustle all day and make dinner for everyone at the end of it all with a clean house to relax into.

I felt like such a mess. Everything was a mess. The house was a mess, my grades were a mess, and with the few lessons I did agree to take on again, I was never prepared at all. I felt like I lost my edge, and began to doubt everything I thought was true about myself.

But wait! I had to ask myself, *what* is *true about any of that? Is this really what failing looks like?*

My kids were happy. They were glad to be back at school. Everyone was fed; my husband stepped up to prepare most, okay all, of our dinners and supported me one hundred percent. So then, what was it, really?

At base, I realized I needed to mother in *my way*, whatever my way looked like. However, that was seen from the outside; it *did not matter*. The job never defined me. The number of hours I spent doing it didn't define me. I had to let it go.

It was an endless cycle in my mind. I constantly felt that I could never do enough each day, while I also worried I was doing too much, terrified about the children, like the proverbial helicopter mother. I could guilt myself into a paper bag.

If I am not a teacher *for my children, who am I? If I can't do everything I think I should as a mother, what kind of mother am I?*

The answer was simple but not so easy to accept. I was afraid I wouldn't be accepted for being myself, that I had to be the music teacher to be seen by others with approval. I couldn't let others know the depth of my inner spiritual world, especially my Christian friends, because I was afraid I was too *woo-woo*. People were going to judge me, judge the way I appeared, what I believed, how I raised my children, and how I earned a living.

You know what, I realized, *they are going to either judge or accept you anyhow! So why not live your life fully for yourself?*

Live authentically, I heard my internal voice say.

I leaped and made a conscious decision to shift my perception, to look at my*self*, from what I thought I was supposed to be to what *could be possible.* It was a sort of revelation and a shedding, like a creature that sheds its skin during a molt.

It's a slow and gradual change to recognize how you used to operate based on old belief patterns and consciously choose new ones. Each day presents an opportunity to make new choices and release the guilt you've built into yourself from years of trying to be someone you're not while learning to embrace who you are. That is why it is referred to as the *unfolding of the self.* When you go inward, look at who you are, you can find an opportunity to love the rawest form of yourself as you need to.

The beauty in this process is that each time I was faced with a choice to do things the old way—how I thought I was supposed to be—or to choose in such a way that felt true to my being, I naturally came out of that protective shell I created.

The world can finally see me because I'm standing in full authenticity. I found that the choices became easier when they were aligned with my core being. The women around me also felt comfortable letting down their guard and being their authentic selves. It's contagious—women living their lives and simply being themselves without fear of judgment or guilt. This is a ripple, and it's creating waves that are part of the inevitable process that is changing our world.

THE TOOL

THE ART OF LETTING GO

Often, when you're told to "just let it go," the phrase incites a visceral reaction.

How could I possibly just let it go!?

Perhaps you were wronged and want validation.

Maybe you have put effort into something or someone. Letting go feels like giving up.

You want to see the thing through, whether it be a project or a relationship, and you have become blind to what it's doing to you.

It's time, now. Stop and reflect.

What is one thing aggravating you? Maybe it's just slightly irritating, or perhaps it's consuming most of your thoughts.

It's probably the first thing you thought of, whether you want to agree right now or not.

Now take that thing, situation, relationship, or job, whatever it may be, and place it in front of your mind's eye, outside of yourself. Close your eyes, and see it, just there beyond arm's reach. How does it make you feel?

List the feelings. Write them down on paper.

What are all the thoughts and ideas attached to this thing, person, or situation?

List those, too. Write them down.

Now, as you look at what you have written, ask yourself: is this how you think you're *supposed* to feel about it, or is it how you *really* feel? Revise your list.

Sometimes we often get caught up in the dream of what could be and not the reality. It's okay. We all do it. We all have desires.

Reread your list. Did you leave out the things you don't want to feel or think?

The thoughts and feelings that you tell yourself you shouldn't have about this?

List those, too.

This list is for your eyes only. It is a safe place, and it's simply a piece of paper. You can even burn it later if you want to. Write until there is nothing left to write about.

The object of this exercise is to truly determine if you're living the reality best suited to you. Please go ahead and read that again—the reality best suited to you.

Your life is your own. From the outside you may think that if you just did this one thing or could make this one relationship work, you will have made it. Maybe you think you will gain the recognition of a person who appears to have got it together, even if that's only in your mind. The thing is, your life is not a cookie-cutter of the person next to you. You were never designed to live life just like your neighbor. And keeping up with the Joneses is a miserable trap.

You must find your own way, your *personal way,* the way that feeds your true purpose, and the energy that will light you up.

This is what it looks like to be living in alignment with your divine purpose.

Now back to your list. If your list no longer brings you anything but happiness and satisfaction, it's time to let it go.

We tend to resist change. Change can be hard. Sometimes we fear it.

But you'll never know what will fill the space that thing is currently taking up in your life until you allow the change.

Make a choice because you love yourself. *Let it go.* Let it go with love and gratitude for bringing you to this place of better understanding yourself. Be gentle with yourself as you go through the process. It's not easy to break these cycles.

It's time.

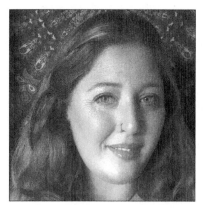

Layne Eliese Mills is a wife and mother to three young boys. She and her family live on the Big Island of Hawaii in their off-grid home that they built themselves while always looking forward to the next big adventure ahead. Layne graduated from Colorado Mesa University with a Bachelor of Arts in Music and studied various forms of spiritual practices such as divination with tarot, palmistry, astrology, the study of the Akashic records, world religions, and theology in her own time for 20 years. After the birth of her third child, she began to pursue offering her knowledge professionally in 2020.

Her passion is in guiding others, especially women and mothers, on a journey to find their true authentic selves and the magic they hold inside and curate a life in full alignment with the way their souls are wired and designed.

You can find out more about Layne's programs and work with her to find your unique mothering design at:

On her website:

msha.ke/layne.eliese.star.spirit

Telephone: (808)769-7197

On Facebook:

https://www.facebook.com/layne.eliese.mills

https://www.facebook.com/LayneStar/

On Instagram:

https://www.instagram.com/LayneEliese

CHAPTER 7

JUST BE A TREE

WHEN IN DOUBT, MEDITATE IT OUT

Michele Tatos

MY STORY

"I have too many tools to help me with life's most challenging moments." Said nobody. Ever.

I'm in my standard soccer-mom gray minivan, driving home with my sweet angels in the back seat, ages two-and-a-half and three. A repetitive song from a recent mommy-and-me music class is blaring, while at the same time, *I am the worst mom ever,* is stuck in a loop in my head.

I'm taking slow deep breaths to calm my racing heart. The nervous sweat is starting to sneak out, a knot has formed in my gut, and I might be on the verge of a silent but deeply defeated and heartfelt cry. I'm clearly overreacting, but my children's first day of preschool was not at all how I fantasized it would be. One of the preschool teachers kindly explained that my son had quite a bit of separation anxiety and did not have a good time—at all. My daughter heard his very loud and continuous distress cries and asked if she could please go into the next classroom to calm him, which the teachers allowed because they were that desperate. My children were only seven months apart, but only one of them enjoyed their first day.

Only one of them appeared to be ready for this new adventure. Where did I go wrong?

Well, despite what we tend to believe, mothers aren't to blame for everything that goes wrong with our children. Each person deals with new situations differently, and stress and anxiety come with being human.

Flash forward 12 years.

"Hey guys, I'm thinking about writing a chapter for a book called Strong Mothers. I want to write about the personal energy management tools I've been using with you both, but I might have to use some personal examples of when you both had challenging times. Would that be too embarrassing?" I blurt out as I enter our living room.

Contemplative pause.

"The tools have helped me, so you should share them, Mom," answers my extremely confident, funny, sweet 13-year-old son, Dax, who is currently lounging on the couch in his soccer uniform with his bruised and muddy knees on display.

"You can talk about how I used to cry in my class after experiences with my PE teacher, and how grounding out the negative energy so I didn't have to dump on my friends at lunch helped me through it." This came from Zaya, my creative, fiery, kind, and empathic 14-year-old daughter, radiating the teenage rebel vibe in her torn jeans, heavy black eye makeup, and bright red curly hair in a wild ponytail.

And just like that, I decided to write this chapter to share my journey from that stressful first day of preschool to where I am today with two amazing and grounded teenagers.

Our life, to be clear, is far from drama-free. Having tools doesn't mean you will suddenly cruise through life without any bumps. We definitely have our fair share. Life is about learning and growing from those bumps. Having tools helps you survive life's big challenges with less collateral damage. They can be a lifeline to hold on to when things are really tough. Providing tools for our children gives them a tiny bit of control amidst the whirling chaos of life.

After that non-stellar first day of preschool, I decided I needed a little meditative mommy time-out to figure out how to support my kiddos on their second day of preschool.

I sneak into my bathroom and close the door. *Every mom with young children hides in the bathroom when they need a second to pull it together, right?*

So, fingers crossed that my angel-pies don't barge in on me, I'm stealthily situated in my bathroom. My eyes are closed; I'm focused on my breath and on calling all my attention back to me. I begin to visualize strengthening my grounding connection to the earth and releasing all my accumulated motherly guilt and stress. And voila! Just like that, I knew what I needed to do! I had to provide my preschoolers with tools similar to the ones I was using at that moment. Why wait?

Why can't I start teaching my kids to meditate? I wish I had known about this magic earlier in my life. I didn't start learning about meditation and personal energy management until I was 30 years old!

Okay. Great! Now I have a plan. The next day, as I was driving my kiddos to school, I went for it. "Hey, cuties, how about we play a fun and creative game on the way to school? Look out the window and pick out your favorite tree as we're driving. Once you have one picked out, close your eyes and pretend you are that tree. Imagine you're big and strong and have roots that go all the way to the center of the earth." They each chose very different trees. One was a huge, beautiful Eucalyptus tree, and the other was a glorious blooming Magnolia tree. Neither child hesitated. They just chose a tree and jumped into the make-believe.

"Now that you are this amazingly strong tree let's pretend you have a super-cool shiny bubble around you keeping you safe and happy. Nothing bad can come into this bubble, and it's filled with smiles and giggles. It can look however you want it to look. It can even be like a Jedi force shield." My daughter had every color imaginable on her bubble, and she added pictures of me, her dad, and her best friend. My son went with the Jedi idea. It was incredible how easily they took to this visualization and how much they enjoyed sharing out loud what they created in their minds.

Hey, maybe I'm on to something! We began a ritual of doing this every day on our way to preschool. I began teaching my children the personal energy management basics of grounding and shielding through guided meditation. *Wow, and yay!*

Here are some quick definitions of Personal Energy Management, Grounding, and Shielding.

Personal energy management means you're consciously choosing how you expend your physical, emotional, mental, and spiritual energy. It's an awareness of how your thoughts, words, and actions impact you and those around you.

Grounding is defined as calling your attention back to your immediate surroundings, anchoring into present time, calming emotions and thoughts, and getting in touch with your internal and external worlds. Grounding can help manage overwhelming feelings or intense anxiety and can help you to be more focused and engaged. One of my favorite mantras is, "Be a tree. Be here. Be now."

Shielding is the process of defining your personal boundaries. When you walk into a room of people who are angry, scared, or sad, you often begin to feel their emotions as if they're your own. Shielding protects you from taking in other people's emotions and negative feelings. Shielding also keeps your emotions to yourself. I still yell, "Shields up everyone!" when my family and I are heading into a crowded event.

Grounding and shielding exercises are also a great way to introduce meditation. Everyone seems to agree that meditation is good for you, but not everyone knows how fun and easy it can be to teach young children.

"Mommy, I'm still awake. Can you read us another book?" Who hasn't heard this a million times? Since the grounding and shielding visualization worked so well, I thought I would play around with some centering and sleepy-time meditations. Why not?

"How about instead of another book, I take you on a fun sleepy-time adventure? Close your eyes and start to listen to the sound of your breath. Now, imagine that a magical animal friend joins you and you both sprout wings and fly over a sparkling rainbow and end up in a peaceful and magical land." This is how it usually started, and then we went to new, fantastical places.

Many nights they wanted to return to certain places they loved. A favorite was a forest with superhero meerkats they could run around and play with. They picked their favorite imaginary meerkat to bring back to snuggle in bed with them as they fell fast asleep. I'm pretty sure we visited the zoo that day and spent a lot of time in front of the meerkat habitat. As they got older, they'd try to lead their own sleepy time meditations for each other. Talk about adorable.

This simple sleepy time ritual teaches children to get out of the analytical part of their mind, the area that obsessively replays events from the day and enters into their intuitive space, where unconditional love, divine calm, and creativity reside. This is called getting centered. The earlier we connect with and trust our intuition, the better.

"Mommy, my best friend, was mean to me at recess today, and I feel awful!" Aha, this is the perfect opportunity to introduce a way to release negative emotions that can get stuck in our energetic and physical bodies! "Close your eyes and imagine you're putting all your frustration, anger, and sadness into a big red rocket ship or a giant soccer ball," which was my son's preference. "Now, say goodbye to those hurtful emotions and send the red rocket ship or soccer ball far, far, far out into space, where the energy of your emotions can be exploded, and then turned into something happy and beautiful to be showered on the world."

It's never too early or too late to start introducing energy work. One of my fondest memories is being invited to my son's fifth-grade class by his teacher to give a one-hour lesson on mindfulness. *I can't believe I agreed to do this,* I thought, as I sat down in front of a class full of fifth graders. *Are they going even to pay attention? Is this going to be too challenging for them? An hour is a long time.* Some children chose to remain in their seats, but my son and his friends sat cross-legged on the carpet in front of me. My son looked at me and gave me the biggest smile. *Okay, I can do this.*

I was completely floored that day by how open and engaged the class was during the discussion on mindfulness and how easily they closed their eyes and embraced meditation. They visualized being a big, beautiful, and strong tree with roots connected deep into the earth and connected to other trees in their life and within their community. I had them breathe in words like calm, grace, and unconditional love to see how it made them feel. They ran different colors through their body to determine how they reacted to each. After each meditation, they drew what they experienced, heads down, with laser focus on that paper in front of them.

I came back several more times. They visualized sending love to their classmates on Valentine's Day and practiced easing their anxiety before going off to a week at outdoor education. Fifth graders are naturals at meditating. Who knew?

"Hey, Mom, I did energy work with my friends at lunch today," my high school freshman daughter said somewhat casually.

"Really? That's awesome! Tell me about it," I encouraged her.

"Well, I started pulling positive energy and love from the universe into a ball in between my hands. My hands were spreading apart on their own because the ball just started getting bigger and bigger. I just went with it. I took the big ball of positive energy and love and threw it up in the air, and let it shower down on my friends. It felt amazing!" Her enthusiasm shined through in her words.

Talk about a happy mama moment! I've tried to instill a sense of joy and playfulness as part of personal energy management. I also stress the importance of setting a positive, healing intention. Energy work is powerful stuff and needs to be used with love and care. If we teach our children early and often about how everything is energy and connected, they can be more in tune with themselves and the universe around them. One of my favorite quotes is from Albert Einstein, "Everything is energy, and that's all there is to it. Match the frequency of the reality you want, and you cannot help but get that reality. It can be no other way. This is not philosophy. This is physics."

Meditation allows you to experience the profound magnitude and beauty of working with energy. Come on! Let's give it a try!

THE TOOL

This is a selection of my favorite meditations for children eight and above. For younger children, you can use the meditations included in "My Story."

Whenever you start something new, set your expectations accordingly. It may take multiple attempts for your children to start engaging. If their eyes are open and they want to move around, or they want to add or change the meditation, let them! Go with the flow and make this a joyful experience.

BE A TREE - AN ACTIVE GROUNDING MEDITATION

Have your child in a standing position holding a ball in their hands. The ball should be a tennis ball or a small softball.

As you read the meditations below, take your cue from your child for an appropriate pace. Speak slowly and clearly and pause to let them experience the feel of the ball or the feel of their breath.

- Close your eyes and notice the ball you have in your hands.
- Start to pass the ball back and forth between your hands.
- Pay attention to how the ball feels on your skin when passing it back and forth.
- Does the ball feel rough on your skin? Does it feel smooth? Does it make your skin tingle?
- Is the ball making any noise as you pass it back and forth?
- Now, keep passing the ball back and forth between your hands, but start noticing how you're breathing.
- Notice how your chest rises and falls as you breathe in and out.
- Breathe in through your nose and out through your mouth.
- Notice the soft noise you make in your nose and mouth as you breathe in and out.
- With your next few breaths, imagine that you are breathing in calmness and unconditional love.
- Each breath fills you with a sense of calm and the feeling of being loved.
- Let that calming and loving breath fill you from the top of your head to the very bottoms of your feet.
- Move your shoulders and your legs and feel how relaxed you are.
- Now, bring your attention to your feet.
- Notice how the ground feels on the bottoms of your feet.

- Move your feet up and down and notice how connected you are to the ground.
- Now, imagine that you are a tree and have roots growing from the bottom of your feet, all the way to the center of the earth.
- Let those roots become even bigger and stronger until you feel that nothing can knock you over.
- Now, start moving your shoulders and your arms and legs.
- Notice the sounds in the room.
- Notice the ball in your hand.
- With your next breath, open your eyes and be back in this room.

CENTERING AND SHIELDING MEDITATION

- Close your eyes.
- Take slow, deep breaths in and out.
- Notice how your chest and stomach go up and down as you breathe in and out.
- Breathe in through your nose and out through your mouth.
- Notice the soft noise you make in your nose and mouth as you breathe in and out.
- With your next breath, imagine that you are breathing in unconditional love and a feeling of complete calm.
- Let it flow from the tippy top of your head to the bottoms of your feet.
- Imagine that you can see a beautiful sparkling golden bridge in your mind.
- Now, pretend that you are walking or running across that bridge into a calm and loving place that is full of yummy-smelling flowers and peaceful trees.
- A gentle breeze is blowing, and you feel the warm sun helping you feel even more relaxed and calm in this beautiful place that is just for you.

- Now, pretend that you have a big, beautiful bubble around your body.
- It is made up of your favorite colors.
- Let your bubble sparkle and shine!
- Inside the bubble, you are safe and happy.
- Nothing bad can get inside this bubble.
- Mean words bounce right off your bubble and never reach you.
- Imagine that your bubble is full of the same calming and loving energy that your body is filled with.
- Now, start moving your shoulders and your arms and legs.
- Notice the ground under your feet and the sounds in the room.
- With your next breath, open your eyes and be back in this room.

I encourage you to join your children in meditating. Being a mom is hard! We could all use some deep breaths and healing visualizations. Record your voice or listen to an app while snuggling with your cuties. There are many great meditation apps available.

If you have the time and energy, reading a meditation to your child can be a truly peaceful and healing experience for both of you. Once you get into the swing of it, you can start making up your own meditation adventures, and then it is beyond awesome!

Take a deep breath, and jump in. When in doubt, meditate it out!

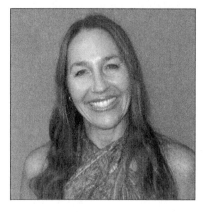

Michele Tatos believes in the power of personal energy management and the magic of meditation! She is the first to say that you are never too young or too old to embrace these life-altering tools.

Michele has been providing energy rebalancing consultations and guided meditations for more than twenty years. Her work focuses on aligning and harmonizing the energy body and chakras while providing you with the information and tools to rebalance and heal yourself.

She spent the first 15 years of her adult life serving in the mental health field in San Francisco, including a position as CEO of a mental health employment agency. She then embarked on a ten-year inspirational journey, working for a nonprofit that served individuals of all ages with developmental disabilities.

Michele would describe herself as an extremely social introvert whose core passions include spending time with her family, spoiling her miniature schnauzer and two bearded dragons, playing soccer and tennis (and someday golf if her husband has his way,) hiking, meditating, and reading science fiction books. Her education includes an MBA, many psychology courses, and more than 20 years of energy and intuition training.

She has had the pleasure, and the chaos, of raising two amazing children who are only seven months apart. Synchronicity at its finest! A planned adoption and surprise pregnancy all at once. Since day one, it has been apparent that these two spirits were meant to be siblings.

In her spare time, Michele enjoys a variety of fun *mom roles,* including girl scout troop leader, PTA president, and youth soccer and basketball coach.

You can find more information on Michele's practice at her website: beatreewithme.com.

CHAPTER 8

LOST AND FOUND

HEALING POSTPARTUM DEPRESSION

Kandi Leigh

MY STORY

I slammed the car door shut, looked at my watch, and glared at John. *Of course, we're going to be late. Again. And it's Christmas Eve!*

I looked at the gifts with their crooked bows and uneven sides. My stomach dropped, and I could already hear the jokes about my subpar wrapping skills. John drove as I signed the Christmas cards for Mom, William, and his wife. The uneven pavement and my frustration made my scribbles even harder to read than usual.

I looked at John. "I really wanted Christmas Eve to feel special." I sighed. "Maybe next year." I paused, then yelled. "And when am I going to take a pregnancy test?"

John's eyes became saucers. "You're only a couple of days late. Let's not start a bad habit."

We had only been trying for a month, so it did seem unlikely I would get pregnant so quickly. But, everything felt *different*. I loved watching moms push their strollers through the mall as a little girl. I never once questioned if I'd be a mother one day. I just knew I would have my own little girl.

John and I continued to argue as he drove, which was not normal for us. He finally pulled into a pharmacy so I could buy a pregnancy test. When we got to my brother's house, John immediately pulled me into the bathroom.

"I wasn't planning to take it here! The focus should be on Anne and William and my new nephew."

John said, "We bought the test. We're taking it now."

A few minutes later, a faint second line appeared on the pregnancy test applicator.

"Ummm, maybe we should have Anne look at it," John said. "Just to be sure." Anne's a nurse.

I opened the bathroom door. "Anne! Can you come here?" She came into the tiny hallway bathroom, took one look at the test, and hugged me. "Wow! Congratulations!"

As I walked out of the bathroom, pregnancy test in hand, William stood there with his video camera covering half of his face. He loved videoing all of our special occasions.

"What's going on?"

"I'm going to have a baby!"

Suddenly, this was the most special Christmas Eve of all.

Eight months later, I was swollen like a balloon. I chatted with Mom on the phone. "Are you sure you're ready for this?" she asked.

"Umm, Mom, I think it's a little late to be asking that question. Does anyone ever really know if they're ready to have a baby?"

"I suppose not," she said.

Thankfully, my pregnancy was easy, and giving birth two months later was almost easier. My little girl, Sarah, shot right out of me.

Life was never the same again.

When I was 17, I had a breast reduction, so I knew there was a chance breastfeeding would be difficult for me. But, I felt the milk come in and saw it dripping from my nipples. I assumed everything was normal. Sarah met the weight requirements to leave the hospital, and off we went.

Two days later, I hadn't slept more than 30 minutes at a time. I wasn't sure who was crying more, Sarah or me. No one prepared me for how hard it would be to set her down just to use the bathroom and take a sitz-bath. And laying her in her crib at night? *Forget it.* She let out blood-curdling screams that made my entire body freeze.

And when she finally dozed, I lay in bed, exhausted, my mind spinning. My body wouldn't relax. I froze when I heard the cry I was already anticipating.

I finally caved. I put Sarah in bed with me to nurse her and let her fall asleep, but she only nursed for a minute before passing out. I tried to sleep too. Ten minutes later, she woke up crying. I tried nursing her again. After a few minutes, she passed out.

This vicious cycle lasted a couple more days until it was time for her follow-up appointment with the pediatrician.

"How's it going?" the young doctor asked. "Is she eating well? Do you have her on a sleep schedule yet?"

My stomach clenched. "Sleep schedule?" I almost cried. I bet she didn't have kids yet. "Not even close. Sarah nurses for a few minutes, passes out, wakes up screaming, and then we start all over."

The doctor weighed her. She was the same weight as when we'd left the hospital.

"Hmm, she should be gaining weight by now. And you need to have her on a feeding and sleep schedule. I need you to come back the day after tomorrow so we can weigh her again."

I cried the entire drive home. How was I going to do this?

A couple of days later, Sarah still hadn't gained weight, and I still wasn't sleeping. Thankfully, Mom took a week off from work to help me. When she walked into my house the first morning, Sarah was crying. I walked into the kitchen holding my tiny daughter with tears in my eyes. I handed the crying bundle over to Mom and said, "I can't stay awake anymore," and walked off. I had no idea what Mom would do, but I felt like it was no longer safe for me even to hold Sarah.

I got in bed. My mind started spinning, and my heart was racing as I listened to Sarah cry for another minute. And then there was silence. After a few minutes, I got my body to relax. I didn't wake up for at least two hours. When I woke up, there was silence. I panicked. *Is Sarah okay? What has Mom done to her?*

I walked into the kitchen and saw Mom snuggling Sarah in her arms, who was fast asleep.

"Mom, how did you do that?"

"I don't know. I just put a pacifier in her mouth and cuddled her up. She fell asleep."

I started crying. I was frustrated because I had hoped not to use pacifiers. But, I was relieved because I had slept, and Sarah had, too.

Friday afternoon, as Mom packed up to leave for the final time, a dam broke loose in me. I sobbed. About three minutes after Mom left, I received a text from Anne. *If you're crying and scared now that your Mom is gone, I promise that's normal.*

I smiled through my tears. For the first time since coming home with Sarah, something felt normal.

Even though the next day was Saturday, John and I had to take Sarah to the doctor to be weighed. Her weight remained the exact same every time we went. Until she gained weight, we had to keep having her checked every other day.

As we got into the car, my body filled with panic. *Would they keep telling me I was doing everything wrong?* We still didn't have a good eating or sleep schedule. Sarah was still latching on to my breast, nursing for about ten minutes, and then passing out. Any little noise would wake her, and she would screech like she was in pain, rooting for my breast. She would latch on again, and then I could feel her falling into sleep as her clenched gums slid off of my chapped nipple. Sometimes I would cry out in pain, which would wake her up.

A couple of nights later, Sarah was crying, seemingly hungry after nursing, and I was crying out of exhaustion and panic. John made a bottle out of some formula we were given at the hospital.

As soon as he stuck the warm bottle in Sarah's mouth, she chugged it. And when she finished the bottle, she cried, wanting more. We gave her a little more, and she immediately spat it up. Her belly was full, but babies can't tell the difference between hunger, gas, or bellyache pain.

The next day, I finally did what I was too scared to do: I called the lactation specialist and explained Sarah's cycle of eating and falling asleep on my breast. The specialist told me to start pumping my breasts for milk right after Sarah eats. She said I should expect to get about five ounces from each breast.

That evening, I figured out how to set up my double breast pump and turned it on. Milk barely trickled from my breasts. After 20 minutes, I pumped maybe half of an ounce.

I cried.

My baby wasn't getting enough food from me. *No wonder she was eating and passing out. Getting the milk out of my breast was exhausting her.*

The next day we took her to the doctor. I held my breath as they set her on the scale. She gained weight!

"We fed her a bottle last night," I told the older doctor, who thankfully was gentler than the first pediatrician.

Dr. Alex placed his hand on my shoulder. "Mom, how are you feeling about bottle feeding?"

I felt tears sting my eyes. He was asking if I was okay with bottle feeding in a world dominated by breastfeeding-only stigmas.

"My baby is gaining weight. I can't believe I didn't know she wasn't getting enough food from me. I'm so relieved she's finally getting what she needs," I said.

I hoped our feeding nightmare was over, but a whole new cycle began. When we gave Sarah her bottle, she chugged it down and demanded more. There was no way a newborn needed 12-16 ounces at a time. And she always proved us right by spitting up what seemed like a lot of fluid.

We tried different bottles and formulas, and the result was always the same. I dreaded feeding her because I knew she would scream, wanting more, and then spit up everywhere.

Soon, it was Christmas Eve again. This time we were celebrating at Mom's house. I was in my kitchen with Sarah's diaper bag feeling panicked as we got ready to leave. I hadn't taken Sarah anywhere besides the doctor. How much formula did I need? How many bottles? How much water? *How would I ever figure all of this out?*

There was a crowd when we got to Mom's house. My dad and my stepmom joined us so everyone could enjoy the grandkids. My nephew toddled around, smiling through his chunky cheeks and playing with anyone who would give him attention.

Sarah cried. *A lot.*

I finally took her into a quiet bedroom to calm her, and this was how we spent most of Christmas Eve.

At the time, I didn't understand how sensitive she was to energy and that being around a crowd of people was overwhelming to her. Christmas Eve became the first of many times we visited family or friends, and I had to sit in a quiet room with her, alone.

A few months later, Sarah was continuously sleeping in bed with us. And I still wasn't sleeping. Sometimes I worried I would roll over on her. Mostly, I just couldn't shut my brain off. *This was normal, right?* Eventually, Sarah began a routine of waking up in the middle of the night and using the bed's headboard to pull herself to standing and then using the bed as a trampoline.

After several nights of her midnight jumping escapade, I got out of bed and found John in the kitchen. It was Sunday morning, and I was supposed to be getting ready for church. I just looked him in the eyes and said, "I'm not okay." And then I went back to bed and cried.

Sarah's birthday was in August, and we decided to celebrate at the beach. We took Mom with us so I could try to rest and relax a little. On the fourth night, John and I went on a date. As we sat and talked without interruption and a crying baby, I felt more like myself than I had in a year. After months of carrying anxiety in my body, I hadn't realized how intense it was until I gave myself space to relax. I just thought I was going through the normal first year of motherhood.

But what I was experiencing, while common, was not normal.

Ten years later, as John and I were on the brink of divorce, I began working with a reiki master teacher. On the day of my first session, John and I had a huge fight. As Mary did reiki on me, I felt a warmth and a vibration I never felt before. As I left, I felt like I was wrapped in a cocoon. My mind felt clearer. I felt like I could breathe for the first time in a long time.

As I continued visiting Mary, I knew I wanted to learn Reiki. It felt like a magical tool, and I thought the whole world could benefit from it. I sailed through Reiki I and Reiki II. In preparation for my Reiki III master retreat, I had to do practice sessions. My friend Carrie recently gave birth for the first time. She was struggling with postpartum depression, and her baby cried a lot. She gave me permission to do distance reiki on both of them.

That session changed my life. Feeling the energy of a newborn baby was the most beautiful energy I ever experienced. I knew I wanted to be able to do more of this. As I worked on the baby, I could hear him saying, "I love you, Momma." Sensing his energy and being able to share that message with Carrie, who was terrified she was a terrible mom, was a huge gift for both of us.

I've been practicing Reiki since 2018 and learning many other tools to help clear, balance, and ground my energy. I now look back on my first year as a mother and realize I didn't have to suffer from postpartum depression. I just didn't have the tools I needed to help me feel better. I honestly didn't know I was allowed to feel good. Being a new mom was scary. It felt like everywhere I turned, there was a message telling me I was making the wrong choices. I kept thinking, *What if this is the choice that ruins my daughter's life?*

I often remind myself that I didn't know then what I know now, and I forgive myself for not connecting to Reiki and meditation sooner. But also, I cheer myself on for being in a space where I can share these gifts with others. One of my mottos in life is to be the person I needed *when.* I now have a tool that I give to new mothers to help them clear, balance, and ground their energy as they spend their days nursing and rocking their baby. But, this is also a beautiful tool for anyone to use at any time during the day to re-center and feel better.

THE TOOL

Two of the most valuable resources a person can use to move blocked energy and keep the energy flowing through the body are water and breathing. The Earth is approximately 70% water, and our bodies are approximately 70% water. This element is freely given and represents our connection to our Spirit and higher self. Drinking water and being properly hydrated are important.

The breath is another way we connect to Spirit, and considering air is freely given, and we breathe involuntarily, I consider it a highly undervalued tool. Although we breathe involuntarily, we (mostly) get to control how we breathe.

The more deeply you breathe, the more ability you have to clear stagnant energy from the body and call in higher vibrational source energy. This can help you de-stress and feel soothed or relaxed and help you feel safer in your body.

When doing breathwork, I breathe in pairs. The first breath carries the intention to clear lower vibrational energy from the body. The second breath carries the intention to call in higher vibrational source energy. Any time we declutter energy from the body, energy will always fill its space, so I recommend being intentional about the energy you refill your body with.

This breathing exercise is based on sacred geometry. You breathe through each of the body's main seven chakra points (energy centers) twice. The chakra points are the crown at the top of the head, the third eye in the center of the forehead, the throat, the heart in the center of your chest, the solar plexus at the bottom of your rib cage, the sacral below your belly button, and the root at your tailbone area. When you breathe, you breathe in for five seconds, hold for five seconds, then release for five seconds. You have two options: you can breathe through each chakra point twice in a row or breathe through each chakra point one time and then breathe through each chakra point a second time. I recommend playing with it and seeing which feels best to you.

If you'd like to see a graphic of the chakras or practice this breathing technique with me, visit the resources page on my website.

There's another tool I'm sharing with you on my resource page that I began using once both of my kids were in school to help them learn to balance and protect their energy, especially while at school. This tool has proven to be a fun way for me to bond with my children in the morning and create more peaceful days. I finally feel like the mother I always dreamed I would be. This tool also helped my daughter connect more to her true self, allowing her to blossom while becoming a teenager, and we finally have a relationship that's better than I imagined it could be.

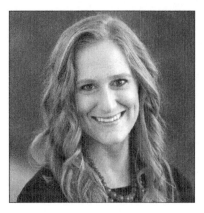

Kandi Leigh is a Reiki Master, hypnotist, intuitive energy reader, and spiritual coach. She offers holistic healing practices and guidance to help people find peace, joy, and balance. She also loves using Tarot and Oracle cards to help provide guidance. One of her strengths is explaining things to people in a way that makes sense to them, being a translator of sorts, and helping people discover tools to help them lead more balanced healthier lives. She loves to help people feel good.

Kandi was first exposed to Reiki as a teenager. In 2015, her brother passed away from pancreatic cancer, and her grief recovery led to learning more about holistic healing arts and discovering who she truly is, what her soul purpose is, and how to live it. As she re-connected to Reiki, she realized her psychic senses were opening up and became filled with awe-like wonder at how amazing energy work truly is. She now thrives in assisting others on their journeys to discovering their gifts and finding their true selves.

She calls herself a true Sagittarius who loves to express her creativity through photography and dance. She grew up in a family of cloggers, traveling all over the US performing from the time she could stand up until she was 14. Since 2010, she has been a wedding, corporate, and lifestyle photographer. Her current passions are shooting elopements in the Smoky Mountains of East Tennessee, where she calls home and shooting 360-degree lifestyle portrait sessions that provide a fusion for family-oriented entrepreneurs.

Connect with Kandi:

On her websites:

http://kandileigh.com

http://holisticwellbeingwithkandi.com

http://kandileighphoto.com

On Facebook: https://www.facebook.com/the.kandi.leigh

Facebook Group: https://www.facebook.com/ascendwithkandi

On Instagram: https://www.instagram.com/the.kandi.leigh/

CHAPTER 9

EVERYDAY ALCHEMY

HOW TO TRANSMUTE TRAUMA AND TRANSFORM NEGATIVE ENERGY

Angela Medway-Smith, Cariad Spiritual,
Life & Soul Alignment Coach

"Your children are not your children.
They are the sons and daughters of Life's longing for itself.
They come through you but not from you,
And though they are with you yet they belong not to you.
You may give them your love but not your thoughts,
For they have their own thoughts.
You may house their bodies but not their souls,
For their souls dwell in the house of tomorrow,
which you cannot visit, not even in your dreams."

~Kahil Gilbran, The Prophet

MY STORY

". . .and then they took us to a French school, all my friends thought I was lucky not having to eat their food," she laughed, eyes shining, a huge grin on her face, her father and brother, sitting on the floor next to her, smiling in adoration.

"Then we went on a boat along the River Seine to the Eiffel Tower!" Her eyes were like saucers now, and she exuded joy and wonder. "It was huge, amazing, and it's much bigger than you think it's going to be. . . now then," she continued excitedly, "I have presents!"

She started rummaging in her suitcase, strewing clothes untidily over the living room floor.

In that pause, my mind was transported to one week earlier. Tears started pouring down my face, and I smiled haplessly through them at my little girl.

"What's wrong, Mammy?" A frown of concern spread over her face. My husband touched my knee. He knew what I was thinking.

"I'm just so happy for you, baby," I replied. I was really happy and relieved. My whole being relaxed as the tears flowed. "Let's see these presents and I'll go and organize dinner. You must be starving."

A few minutes later, I was in my kitchen proudly wearing an apron with a cat wearing a beret waving a French flag. I pulled the vegetables from the fridge and started peeling and chopping.

More tears flowed. My body was wracked with sobs as the images from the last week played back in my mind. *It's fine. They can't hear you. Just let it go,* I heard a voice say as I called in the power of the violet flame and let the pain and trauma flow away with my tears.

I'm used to hearing voices; I'm psychic, clairvoyant, clairaudient, and clairsentient. Spirit, my guides, angels, and the ascended masters have been talking to me like this for as long as I can remember; most of the time, I listen. "Don't tell anybody, Angela; they won't understand," my grandmother told me when I was a little girl.

One Week Earlier

3 am. I sat up in bed with a start. A voice said, *Wake up! Something's wrong!* My husband was fast asleep beside me, breathing peacefully. *No. He's fine. It's Caitlin!* said the voice.

I ran into my daughter's room, where she lay in a pool of vomit, eyes sunken, face ashen. "Mammy, can't breathe. It hurts Mammy." She stammered, every breath an effort, her face soaked in tears.

I lifted the dirty sheets away from her. "Let's get you sorted, baby." I pulled her blood glucose meter from the nightstand and tested her blood sugar levels. HI, it read. *Shit, over 32, the meter can't read it! I thought.*

"I need to test for ketones, baby, and let's see your insulin pump," I said gently, reaching over. I could see the red light flashing on her pump. The insulin had run out—ketones 3.5, in the danger zone.

Oh my God, it's a hospital if I can't sort this out in half an hour, I thought. "We need to get some insulin into you; let's go downstairs."

We staggered down the stairs, her limp arms draped over my shoulder. "Sit here. I'll get a pan in case you're sick again, insulin, and some water for you. You need to drink."

I administered the insulin, and she winced, "Mammy, it hurts so bad. Can't breathe. Can't breathe."

I'd never seen her this bad before.

Check her ketones again. Now! Then phone the hospital, said the voice.

Ketones 8—way into ketosis. *Her organs are shutting down. She'd be in a diabetic coma if I didn't wake up! Please, God. No! How can this be happening so fast!?*

I rang the hospital and told them we were on our way and woke my husband. He needed to get our son to school later. I pulled on some clothes as he put our daughter into the car wrapped in a blanket.

I drove for half an hour, breaking the speed limit, through the sleeping streets, onto the motorway, then a long dark road to the Pediatric Intensive Care Unit in the city hospital.

"Help me, please! I need a wheelchair!" I shouted to a porter.

I pushed the chair while running along the corridor, pretending it was a game, "Wheeeeee! We'll be there in a minute, baby; the doctors will make you better," I told her, despite my heart banging in my chest with fear.

"She's too dehydrated; we can't get a line in; we need to call the consultant," said the doctor. I stroked her hair, "Everything will be okay." I said and shot anxious glances at the nurses and doctor as the ketones climbed.

Ketones 11. *Please God, please God, PLEASE GOD, help them save her,* I prayed silently over and over, like a Novena.

My prayers were answered. A beautiful angel in the guise of a consultant glided in, smiling warmly. Five minutes later, "The line's in, fluid and insulin are flowing nicely. We need to get her into Intensive Care."

I followed behind, hugging her blanket, as her bed was wheeled down the dimly lit corridor into a room of four beds. I scanned the room, three sleeping children of different ages hooked up to beeping machines, keeping them alive and nurses quietly floating silently between them.

"Nothing to do but sit and wait now," said her nurse. I pulled my daughter's blanket over me in the cold plastic chair and reached over to hold her hand.

Of course, there's something you can do, said the voice. I could hear my heartbeat slowing as the panic subsided, my mind stopped racing, and calm descended.

Open yourself as a channel. Call in the angels. All will be well.

I'd trained as a healer many years earlier, but I worked in mental health services while raising my children, healing quietly in the background. I was a Senior Manager now, still hiding the fact I spoke to guides and angels.

I opened my heart and mind, and the energy flowed. Beings of light gathered around the bed as I, now exhausted, drifted into a light sleep, still holding her hand.

The nurses, doctors, and angels worked for three days and nights and slowly brought my little girl's body into balance. Gradually, the limp, lifeless, frightened little girl whose organs were shutting down was transformed back into my bubbly, smart, feisty, caring, independent child.

She said with big eyes smiling on the third day, "Mammy, I can still go to Paris, can't I? I'm fine now."

"Let's see what the doctors say, baby," I replied weakly and terrified. *What if it happens again? How will they cope?* The thought invoked panic in my body, and my stomach lurched.

All will be well; she will be looked after, said the voice.

My heart sank. Another fight began to convince her doctors and her father that all would be well and suppress my strong maternal urge to keep her close, home, and safe.

The trip had been planned for months—care plans, emergency plans, plan A, plan B, plan C; teachers trained, specialists brought onboard, every eventuality considered, planned for; surely she'd be safe.

24 hours later, she was on a bus to Paris. The other mothers cried as they waved off their children; every cell in my body screamed as I smiled and waved, *hold it together, Angela, she will be safe.*

And she was absolutely fine.

My husband and I lost six angel babies before our son and daughter were born. Both were premature, special care babies. I have a host of auto-immune conditions, and they are miracles.

Despite my best efforts, two years of breastfeeding each child, healthy organic diets, late introduction of common allergens into their diets, complementary medicine rather than antibiotics, my daughter still developed a host of auto-immune conditions. My son managed to escape this gene lottery.

Aged three, it was juvenile diabetes that hit. At four, alopecia and she lost her beautiful, long auburn wavy hair. At five she faced psoriasis, so bad her skin bled, and only her hands and feet were clear. And at age nine, she was diagnosed with celiac disease. Every day became a challenge. Simply leaving the house required military planning and preparation.

I fought, ensuring the right support was available in education for her to thrive. I educated teachers, fighting with the local education authority for support at school, so my husband and I weren't called in every day to deal with low and high blood sugars, and so she could learn safely and effectively.

Despite the many challenges we traveled the world, and she was encouraged to be brave and bold and follow her dreams.

My babies are grown now, 20 and 23, and I'm incredibly proud of the amazing humans my husband and I raised. There were other experiences, like the one I've recounted here, and each time we did our best, fighting for our kids, following our intuition, and using common sense. That's all you can do as a parent.

It would have been so much easier to wrap our miracle children up in cotton wool and protect them from the world. But growing balanced, independent humans takes guts, and that means letting go to allow them to make their own mistakes and mature, however scary it feels—teaching them they can do anything if they work for it.

We're stepping out of our fear and becoming strong mothers.

To do this, we need tools to support us at our fingertips. After all, we're only human!

I now work as a life and soul alignment coach, women's retreat leader, spiritual channel, and healing and intuitive development teacher. My soul's path is to empower people with the tools they need to soar—to tap into their intuition, align with their own soul's path, and access the incredible universal energies we have available. We can live our best lives and make the most of this human experience.

We humans unwittingly store negative energy and trauma in our energetic and physical bodies, and not attending to this toxic build-up can create *disease* later.

The tool I'm sharing with you is ancient alchemy you can use in everyday situations to clear this negative energy, transmute trauma, and transform any situation's energy. With practice, you can intend and send this energy to the past, present, or future.

It's practical, alchemical energy and available to everyone.

Welcome to the violet flame!

THE TOOL

"Are You Ready?
This is your time—the time of enlightenment.
You can choose whether to sit,
remain in your current position and be blind to the possibilities,
or embrace them.
As always, it is your choice.
The balance of existing in this human world
or soaring with all the gifts of your spirit are your choices."

~The Ascended Master St. Germain
Channeled by Angela Orora Medway-Smith, in *The Book of Many Colours.*

In simple terms, the highest vibrating form of light is pure, clear light, which is the light of the Creator, the Divine. This light is broken up into a number of divine rays, and each ray represents a different quality of the Divine, their energy presented here on Earth.

Each of these divine rays is overseen by ascended masters, Archangels, or angelic collectives. They hold different energy and have a different purpose; a unique number, name, properties, color, symbol, patron, active principle, and crystal energy that aligns with them.

These energies have been available to mankind for thousands of years and have been written about by the great spiritual channels Helena Blavatsky, Alice Bailey, Aurelia Louise Jones, and others.

I have also been used as a channel by the ascended masters and angelic collectives to demystify the power of the divine rays and bring these practical tools to 21st-century readers in *The Book of Many Colours: Awaken Your Soul's Purpose With The Divine Rays.*

The seventh divine ray and the violet flame are overseen by the ascended master St. Germain (and a host of angels). Its energy is change, transformation, alchemy, clearing, transmutation, self-exploration, and personal change.

I've used it for many years to transmute negative energy and bring about everyday alchemy, and you can do this too!

There are many different ways you can call in the transformational energy of the violet flame:

- Invocation

- Meditation

- Affirmation

- Visualizing yourself, others, or a place bathed in its energy

- Visualizing yourself, others, or a place protected by its sacred symbol

- Programming a crystal to hold this energy by simply holding and intending the energy to flow when you need it

- As healing energy using the Violet Flame Rescue Flames accredited healing system

Each of these different methods will appeal to different people and are good for different situations. I'm going to share with you the invocation and visualization I use to start and end my day; I don't get out of bed without it! I intend that it balances and energetically protects me.

If I rush, jump out of bed and forget, I feel as if I'm wearing the wrong clothes, and nothing feels right until I remember why!

You can use this any time of the day, whenever you want to transmute negative energy.

VIOLET FLAME INVOCATION

Beloved, I AM Spirit bright

Seal me in your tube of light

From Ascended Master Flame

Called forth now in God's own name

Let it keep my Temple free from all discord sent to me.

I am calling forth Violet Fire to blaze and transmute all desire

Keeping on in freedom's name

'Til I am one with the violet flame

Repeat this three times, as you do, visualize yourself being surrounded in a tube of violet light that comes from the Divine, through your soul, through your higher self, and surrounds you in cleansing, clearing energy, transmuting and transforming negative or stuck energy, protecting you in the divine light of the violet flame.

Feel all negative or stuck energy leave your body, returning to Mother Earth to be recycled, repurposed, and reborn.

All energy is neutral; it's up to us how we program it!

You can tap into the energy of the violet flame to transform and transmute negative energy and trauma anytime, anywhere.

I work closely with the ascended master and angelic collectives and am incredibly grateful for the patronage of St. Germain. My work with the violet flame and the other divine rays is extensive.

As my gift to you, I've recorded a meditation with the violet flame for personal and ancestral clearing. You can find this, together with a beautiful print-out of this invocation, at:

https://www.cariadspiritual.com/strongmothers.

I'm passionate about the potential of the divine rays for unlimited energetic support; to help you be more intuitive, more creative, receive healing, motivation, unconditional love, or nurturing energy, create your own miracles, and align with your soul's path.

Find out more about the divine rays in *The Book of Many Colours: Awaken Your Soul's Purpose With the Divine Rays* (Amazon and Barnes & Noble) or https://www.cariadspiritual.com/.

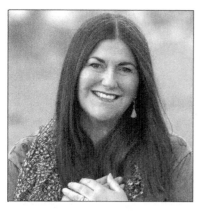

Angela Orora Medway-Smith is a spiritual channel and teacher, master healer, coach, and retreat leader from Wales. Her business is called Cariad Spiritual, and she works both in-person and online spreading the light at workshops, festivals, and retreats all over the world.

Cariad is a Welsh term of endearment derived from *caru* – to love. It reflects who she is, a spiritual being who works from the heart with love. Holistic healing is her passion. Over the years, she's set up healing clinics, created spiritual festivals and holistic events, raised money for children and baby charities, as well as supported hundreds of healers on their path with classes and training and giving thousands of clients worldwide guidance from spirit.

Angela helped found Divine Energy International, a worldwide membership non-profit for energy healers, offering support, training, and many other benefits to our tribe of brave healers. Its vision is *a world where energy healing is for all.* She's on a mission—changing the world one person at a time.

She devotes her life to awakening divine souls like you to their potential. She believes that we all have the ability to transform, to emerge from the chrysalis of this human life, to be the butterfly, and soar. To develop a deep connection to our soul and align with our true destiny. She has developed many different tools in her 35+ years of the spiritual journey to support you to achieve this.

Angela is incredibly blessed to be a direct channel to the Angelic Realms and Ascended Masters and has channeled books on the divine rays and their sacred flames called *The Book of Many Colours* and *The Book of Many Flames* to help people connect to their soul's path through these amazing vibrations and is a co-author of the #1 Amazon bestseller *25 Tools for Goddesses: Volume 4 of the Wellness Universe Ultimate Guide to Self-Care.*

Angela offers spiritual consultations, life & soul alignment coaching, women's retreats, healing, healer, and intuitive development training worldwide.

Connect with Angela at https://www.cariadspiritual.com/

CHAPTER 10

MY MOTHER
WAS KIDNAPPED!

CREATING QUALITY YEARS
FOR LOVED ONES WITH DEMENTIA

Linda Aileen Miller, LMT, CD(DONA)

MY STORY

The night of her passing, within three minutes after I got home, three
pennies dropped onto my kitchen floor
ONE. AT. A. TIME!

Remembering that famous song, *Pennies From Heaven*,
I believe my mother had indeed arrived!

She saved pennies for as long as I can remember
in clear Mason jars, separated by circulation dates.

To her father, she was Kat.
When she married Dad, he called her Kit.
I can still see Kathryn Marie walking the assisted living facility halls
sharing KitKat bars, with red and gold labeled
yummy milk chocolate, on Halloween and Valentines!

May memories of your mom, NanaBobana,
Bingo Buddy, or Queen make you smile, always.

Beautiful, strong mothers live in our hearts forever!

2012, my mother sat rocking in her dark red overstuffed recliner. Hands on her head, crying, she repeatedly asked, "What's wrong with my brain?"

Two falls resulting in head trauma lead me to a possible misdiagnosis— Traumatic brain injury (TBI)/hydrocephalus (water on the brain) versus regular dementia. They often present similarly.

Sometimes in life, the child becomes the mother.

Over-medicated and confused, my kidnapped mom moved south. Together with a new doctor—who had a heart and a brain—we helped her have five better years without dementia drugs.

Family and Thanksgiving were important in our home.

Her assisted living facility didn't allow guests for Thanksgiving; I reserved a private room and took our meal to her. Mom loved it! As we finished, she looked into the garden. Her eyes dropped towards a nearby squirrel, and she softly said, "Maybe we should give him something. He looks hungry."

Mom wanted to feed the world. Feeding at least half of southern rock 'n roll for years was her job! She tried to fix everything, rarely asking for what she needed.

It was important to her to treat people equally, which she learned from her mother. If Grandmommie gave me one dollar, she would do the same for my brother, Chip, and our cousins.

I saw Mom angry three or four times in my life:

1. When I was 15-she shook a broom at me! It was probably well-deserved!

2. When Brian was born, Dad wouldn't leave his hypnosis convention.

3. When I threw away her rotten bananas, she growled!

She smiled when she played six bingo cards while looking across at your numbers and seeing ones you missed! Her wonderful laugh and childlike innocence were with Mom almost until her last breath.

Her greatest joys revolved around all things musical: Chip's and Brian's, Jamie's and Derek's, the Beatles and Diana, MJ and anyone I took her to see in Vegas, and always Elvis!

Music was part of the five days before her passing, 3:33 pm, January 3, 2017. I imagine she found a band or two in Heaven!

Curiously, one day, she listened to nurses having a private conversation with her roommate. Shushing me, she said, "It's my job. I have to make sure she's safe!" She and Sara looked out for each other.

Mom was proud of her family, even though she often said, "Chip's a little stinker!"

She loved her grandson more than life. Anytime she wouldn't take her meds, all I had to say was, "I promised Brian I wouldn't let you be in pain." Boom! Down the hatch!

Teasing her about loving the boys most, she adamantly replied, "No, no, I love you more, but don't tell them!" Then she giggled. Does your mother giggle?

Glowing, she remembered buying Derek Trucks' first guitar when he was eight years old. While I shared a picture of him with her, she pondered. "Now he's an old man! And he's famous?"

Mom wanted to go back to Vegas one more time and to go water skiing and roller-skating.

She forgave everyone no matter what. Rarely did anyone see her cry or hear her cuss! I was lucky. She did both with me.

Dementia, regular or trauma-induced, stole the mother I knew. We learned to make life work through pain and struggles, loving each other deeper, despite or because of it.

Without a doubt, she was the kindest, strongest, sweetest woman God ever created. She loved fiercely and gently. Both were her strengths and her weakness.

I felt angry in 2005 when my brother passed way too young. Three years later, my dad joined him. Then Mom's life changed, and I understood. God in His/Her infinite wisdom gave me the easiest journey.

Seeing her growl when I threw out her brown bananas, I wondered. *How many years had she held that? Good for her!*

Mom taught me two major lessons.

Love. . .no matter what.

Always say thank you.

No matter how hard things got at the end of the day, she always said thank you every day.

When her mind failed, she didn't know who I was. Struggling to remember, she said the most important thing she ever said:

"I'm sorry, I can't remember who you are. My mind is all messed up."

I excused myself and walked out for a minute choking back tears. When I returned, she'd rolled her wheelchair over beside her roommate. They were figuring it out together.

Quietly, as if telling a long-kept secret, she said, *"I do know this. I don't know who you are. I do know I love you more than anything in the whole world and want to thank you for being here!"*

Her heart knew the truth of what her mind could no longer remember.

"This is holy ground. We're standing on holy ground. There are angels all around." Thanks, Geron Davis, for these words*. My momma was one.

It's Christmas
She never said a word.
Most times she wouldn't.
Momma never complained…
Before dementia came
It's how she was raised
It's who she was.
Attending a special dinner
Dressed up in silver and gold
Her tired bent body… still precious
Celebrating life!
Grateful she taught me that!
Looking down at her feet…smiling
I brought out her surprise
Her white rubber Crocs were old.
Sparkling eyes opened the box
Like a child on Christmas morn
Exclaiming, "They're Beautiful!"
New shiny silver shoes!
"Merrills? They look expensive!"
"They were!" I replied
Immediately she looked sad.
"I don't want you spending on me."
"Don't be sad, Mom," I replied.
"Be happy! I spent your money!"
She raised her head and grinned.
"You did? Good!
Go get some for you, too!"
Off we went….
All shiny and sparkling head to toe!
"Merry Christmas, Momma
You were always my best present…
ALWAYS!"

Mom taught us things that will carry on as part of her legacy—one of the cutest from cousin Margaret. She shared the following words with her stretch class, and supposedly the ladies still say them.

"I can shake my shoulders. I can shake my knees. I'm a free-born American. I shake what I please!" And shake they did!

God blessed us all with Miss Kathryn! She was unconditional love! I feel blessed God chose her to be my mom.

And then. . .

She asked if we could call Chip. She wanted him to know she was okay and understood if he was too busy to come to see her.

"Don't you think we should do that? Don't you think we should call Chip? Don't you?" I held her, telling her Chip knew and watched over us from Heaven. The look of shock was heartbreaking. "You mean Chip's gone? When? Why didn't I know that?" She did know. She didn't remember.

Part of my momma died May 24, 2005. Last night another part died all over again. Thanking me for helping her remember, we hugged for a long time. We cried together, again. Dementia is Hell on Earth! Finding ways to cope is Heaven!

BANANA-NANABOBANA. THE SAGA OF BANANAS!

Growling primal guttural sounds…angry, mean, and scowling.

Who is this woman you have found deep inside full of pain and growling?

Where is my mother? What have you done? Why did she go away?

This person I don't know.

I can no longer stay.

I've done my best for three long years.

My days and nights are filled with tears.

Doing things I do know how…

To hold my ground/not fall down

Doesn't matter anymore.

The sadness is profound!

Hers and mine. We try

To be the best of who we are

Dementia is a demon

My Mom's a Superstar!

Who would have thought rearranging furniture could cause such chaos?

Not I!

The charge nurse called earlier that day. "We need to move your mother's bed. It's too hard on my staff to change her at night with the bed against the wall," she said.

Interpretation: "We are short-staffed and/or have hired inept persons."

I said, "The bed has been that way for eight months. It's where she feels safe. It's where she *is* safe. Tucked in, fractured right hip against the wall, with the collage of her family close enough to touch should she awaken feeling alone. I have seen her do it. She cannot roll onto her right hip, fearful she will hurt it. Her fractured right elbow, with two pins from her bicycle accident in 1990, still causes shoulder pain."

Her mind thinks she fractured the shoulder too. She's fearful of anyone touching those spots, crying out in pain if they do. She gets in and out of every bed, rolling on her left side, aided or alone.

Bodies have cellular memory long after our brain forgets.

The nurse says, "I need to move her bed. Putting another alarm on her bed and her wheelchair. There's a mat on the floor beside her right side. Her bed will be parallel, like her roommate's. The left side will be next to the air conditioner. It's a low bed. If she does try to get out, she will not have as far to fall."

I reply, "There's nothing about this I like. It's been the way it is for eight months. It's what works best for her. She likes being tucked against the wall, minimizing her chances of being injured."

I later receive the nurse's voicemail. She moved it anyway.

"Fuck you!" I said into the empty air space. Then I cried. After work, putting on my best game face, I went to see. Mother sat, teary-eyed, at the end of her bed. Her half-in, half-out, dazed-confused blank canvas came earlier today.

I asked how she liked her new bed—the one with the scooped-out mattress sitting a foot from the floor. She replied a bit surly, "I liked the old one just fine. Why did they change it?"

"I don't know, Mom. They thought this would be better." Looking at the big ugly black mat folded up between the bed and nightstand, all I could feel was rage.

She sat staring, defeated, because people changed what felt like her safe corner of the world into someplace she didn't understand. She was angry with me—angry because she thought I had changed it. She "liked it before." She is never angry with staff; that's not who she is; the anger falls on me. It's okay.

Now I will tell you what else I saw...

There was a space wide enough on the left to fall, wedging her between the bed, wall, and air conditioner. It's the side her body knows to turn to. It's what her pattern is! I promise you! She'll try! It's directly next to the air conditioner. She's always cold.

In this configuration, every time someone happens to be present to assist her in or out of bed on the right side, it will cause her emotional angst, frustration, and physical stress. She's very afraid of the "shattered" parts of her.

The saddest thing I saw was her little bed, nearly on the floor. I sat on it. Sitting at the foot end, I was not at eye level with her roommate's bed.

Not even capable of feeling safe myself, having to squat to sit on the edge, using muscles much stronger than hers at 93, I push myself to stand. *How will she do this?* It wasn't equal. It felt wrong.

Guests won't be able to sit beside her bed, gently holding her hand, having a conversation. They'll be bending over, looking down, and awkwardly trying to make it work. There's always the option of sitting on the mat, on the floor, beside the bed.

Late-stage dementia patients are often childlike. They want to be like everyone else. Don't we all?

Are you angry yet?

When understaffed facilities don't answer call lights for thirty minutes or fail to come when she needs to pee, I see my mother falling, attempting to put herself in or out of bed because her brain thinks she can!

I see her falling further because the bed is a foot off the floor, her frail body without support, trying to maneuver independently. Attempting to do what worked for months, her head will now be at the foot of the bed, looking up at the collage of her family. That's what her body memory will do, whether it's logical or not! Dementia doesn't know logic.

If she successfully navigates—by some miracle—from the wheelchair to the bed, there are other problems.

She will feel small.

She will feel different.

She will feel less than, not understanding why her bed is on the floor, not much higher than a pallet.

She will feel disoriented in a space that had some semblance of safety yesterday.

This makes no f-ing sense! It won't be easier to get her in or out, up or down. It won't be easier for staff to get down on the floor to change her during the night. It won't make her feel safer. It certainly won't make me feel my mother is safer. Until the day I die, I won't understand the lunacy behind this decision.

It'll be daylight soon. My heart is heavy, my red eyes swollen, too many tears.

Yet, at dawn's light, somehow stepping up, advocating for her will happen.

When you are the voice for those who have none, it's what you do.

I'm doing my best to get a logical answer. Intuition tells me there's a facility inspection at the core, with precious little about safety for my mother or staff!

I don't believe a fire marshall code had squat to do with this. Firefighters are big, strong, tough guys. They're most capable of getting my mother up and out of bed whether the damn thing is facing north, south, east, or west!

To you, the one who wears the 'in-charge' hat, don't think for a minute that you won. Even after saying I didn't agree, you moved it anyway! So much for patients' rights!

This woman in bed 407-2 is *my* mother! I will fight your egotistical ass to the wall and back to protect her until her last dying breath, or mine! That's what strong women do! You didn't move the furniture. You turned my mother's world upside down. I intend to rock yours!

Two days later, hospice informed me her organs were shutting down.

The nurse stole her hope and her dignity.

And Mom gave up.

Within a week, she left. In her final moments as we lay together, my hand on her heart, her soul touching mine, knowing we both did the best we could.

Because we did!

Much healing has happened since her passing. July 3rd came and went. Thoughts of her popped up. Not once did I think, *Mom passed six months ago today!* Six months! Remembering stories of her life all day, with no notice of the six-month anniversary! Two days later, writing the date, it hit me! Pretty sure that's healing in progress.

Celebrating the 50th anniversary of my 20th birthday was rapidly approaching—the first birth day my mother will not be with me.

There will be no sweet, handwritten message on a Hallmark card. There will be no phone call with her soft southern drawl on the other end of the line. No hugs with a constant gentle pat, pat, on my shoulder. No gifts carefully chosen and perfectly wrapped. No loving, smiling face watching with anticipation for my reaction as I open them. No, "I Love You," "I Love You More," "I Love You Most," laughter like we always shared. For the first time in 70 years, my precious mother won't be physically present on my birth day.

As tears flow like a river, I'm aware there is no doubt she'll show up in her own unique way. Her love will be felt on July 17th, 2017, the day I turn 70!

Thanks, Momma, for all you gave me for seventy years. Most of all, thank you for being born, being my mom, and showing me what *strong mothers* look like even to your last breath.

P.S. Thanks! The pennies continue to fall at just the perfect moment.

I love you more!

THE TOOL

Tools for a strong mother and human are much the same. Lots of them are easy and free! Find what creates 'feel good' warmth like an all-over hug. That creates oxytocin. Oxytocin is our natural drug, filling us with love!

I used many of these tools with my mother. They brought visible change to her cognitive function, emotional outlook, and physical stress.

1. Acupressure, barefoot walks, warm baths, dancing (clothed or naked), massage, meditation, myofascial release.
2. Celebrate life's moments with candles, laughter, music!
3. Listening more than we speak.
4. Patience. All things happen in God's time.
5. Reading or writing a good book.
6. Research! No one has all the answers.
7. Using our voices to advocate.
8. A strong spiritual connection.
9. Always say thank you!

And love. Always love. Waltzing in the moonlight (clothed or naked) with love; all is right with the world!

Thank you!

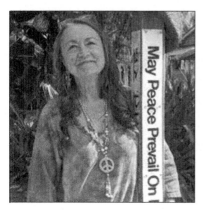

Linda Aileen Miller, LMT, CD(DONA), is a master-level facilitator supporting women, men, and newborns experiencing the mind-body effects of PTSD to heal and live joy-filled. Following a 32-year career with Delta, she retired three trips after 09/11/2001.

Constantly expanding her education, as an expert-level John F. Barnes Myofascial Release specialist, with twenty-four years of experience in holistic bodywork, she is a certified Integrative Breathwork practitioner with roots in Transpersonal Psychology. Linda is also a Level 2 Holy Fire Reiki Master.

In 1969 as an unwed mother-to-be, Linda left her home, family, and friends and moved to Indianapolis. She believed in her heart that offering her child for adoption was her only choice. At the time, it was.

It was a choice that led her to become a doula. Mothering the mother is a sacred privilege in so many ways. "No one should birth or die alone."

An International Certified Birth Doula, and fierce advocate for the unborn, she has extensive training in supporting and holding space for all of life. Linda is currently training with The Institute for the Study of Birth, Breath, and Death and plans to begin teaching Amy Wright Glenn's work in 2022.

A three-time self-published author/poet, Linda collaborated with twenty-four women on her first #1 Amazon bestseller, The Ultimate Guide to Self-Healing, Volume 4, from Brave Healer Productions. She enjoys helping others embrace authentic healing, living filled with peace, love, and balance.

*Thank you, Geron Davis, for the beautiful lyrics to the hymn "This is Holy Ground."

Find her and share at:

Website: lifeisthemuckmagicandmiracles.com

Website: lovingbirthjourneys.com

Email: Linda@lovingbirthjourneys.com

Facebook: https://Facebook.com/LAMLMTMFR/

Facebook: https://Facebook.com/TheInnerJourneyProductionsLLC/

Instagram: https://www.Instagram.com/aileen.linda

CHAPTER 11

LOTUS BIRTH: CORD OF CONNECTION

REJOICE IN YOUR WOMB POWER FOR LASTING VITALITY AND PLEASURE

Lulu Trevena, Artist, Quantum Healer, Soulful Living Coach,
Art of Feminine Presence® Teacher

"Whenever and however you intend to give birth,
your experience will impact your emotions, your mind,
your body, and your spirit for the rest of your life."

~Ina May Gaskin

MY STORY

I stretched my gaze with gentle caressing wholeheartedness across the room to the faces of dear friends who had collected for my fortieth birthday. My heart was a cascade of joy and love. The soft glow of candles flickering on the tables around the room and the calm lake outside the large glass doors held us all in a huge embrace. It was not the 'normal' party of drinking and loud music; it was reverent, exactly what I chose for myself and one that massaged my heart and soul.

My gratitude speech to my guests was sealed as I bowed my body, heart, and head toward the ground in reverence for each of them and the journeys we shared. This night was a self-celebration and a community celebration.

I am a deep, sensitive, feeling, and thinking woman, and in many ways, it has taken me years to love that about myself. I've experienced others less willing to appreciate that about me.

My forty-first year brought another gift into my world, our planned third child to our family. Our first two daughters were both planned home births. In this, my third pregnancy, I explored the practice of lotus birthing. The first time I heard about this method, some ten years prior, it didn't resonate at all. After much exploration, other mothers' experiences, and sincere consideration—including sitting with this style of birth in my meditations—it felt aligned and truly beautiful.

What is a Lotus Birth?

Lotus birth is the practice of leaving the umbilical cord uncut after childbirth so that the baby is left attached to the placenta until the cord naturally separates at the umbilicus. Wikipedia (https://en.wikipedia.org/wiki/Lotus_birth)

Some people choose a lotus birth because they view the placenta as belonging to the baby. Believers in this practice do not see the placenta as a medical by-product but rather an extension of the baby that they feel should disengage independently.

Monroe K, Rubin A, Mychaliska K, Skoczylas M, Burrows H. Lotus birth: A case series report on umbilical nonseverance. *Clin Pediatr (Phila).* 2018;58(1):88-94. doi:10.1177/0009922818806843

While some people cite the lotus flower and its symbolism of unity and rebirth for the name of this practice, it actually comes from events in 1974, when a pregnant California woman named Clair Lotus Day learned about the behavior in chimpanzees and began to question why humans don't do it.

https://www.verywellfamily.com/lotus-birth-4177642

Practitioners of lotus birth claim these benefits: a gentle, less-invasive transition for the baby from womb to the world, increased blood and nourishment from the placenta, decreased injury to the belly button, which is often classed as the first scar or wound on the physical body. The "first relationship" (connection) is the baby and the placenta. (womb & mother)

It was not something I publicly declared or shared with others. I honor all women and celebrate them choosing what is right for their own bodies and those they carry in their wombs. To be empowered by birth. It is very personal. Women's bodies are miraculous and sacred; the birthing process is natural and exquisite. Unfortunately, all too often, it seems to have been defined as a medical procedure.

In my first planned home birth with a professional midwife, we were redirected to a hospital as a precaution in the final stages of labor, which resulted in my choices and the midwife's not being heard. After a non-consensual episiotomy, forceps delivery, and forced placenta removal, I felt violated. I discharged myself and my baby from the hospital two hours later. My midwife cared for us daily like a loving matriarchal figure. There was much healing physically, psychologically, and emotionally after this.

My second daughter was a water birth at home, with an easy, blissful two-and-a-half-hour labor. I'm pre-warning you about my next statement. Birth can be orgasmic. You may have never heard that before! A woman in her power in birthing is powerful, sensual, and divine. She is a Goddess, birthing new life. A woman needs to be sacredly cared for during birth. I advocate for women in this way.

I felt the warm water embrace me as I rocked my body, moving on all fours in the birthing pool. It had a central position in our lounge room, the morning light now streaming in the windows. The assorted candles were slowly melting. The antique sideboard, where they rested with crystals, flowers, and my pregnancy cast in its full bloom, leaned against the wall. Heartfelt gifts from many soul sisters given to me at our Blessingway rested on the lower side table. A Blessingway is a soulful gathering of women to *bless the way* for the baby and mother with awareness and sisterhood.

I have found comfort and strength are sourced from being in environments that allow for safety, freedom, and vulnerability. After all, a naked woman giving birth is as vulnerable as it gets.

Trusting my own guidance and body, I felt the need to get out of the birthing pool and stand. With the support of the midwives and my husband, I continued laboring standing. Grunting, swaying, consciously breathing. Our older two children played nearby. Gravity works well for birthing; standing supports the grand entrance from the body to the air. I placed my hand between my legs and felt the crown of my little one's head. I allowed her to drop into my hands. Our second daughter, Khea, was standing behind me, and as our baby's head emerged, she was facing her. She saw her little face first.

The house was filled with the welcoming of a new soul and family member. My body filled with elation and exhaustion. It was now time for the second stage of labor, delivering the placenta. As in lotus birth, this happens while still attached to the baby. Our older two daughters had a soccer final, so they were bustled off by my husband. My midwives supported me through this second stage. I lovingly lifted our new daughter to my breast and nursed her. The innate effects of breastfeeding can often support the placenta naturally being released. But that was not so. It became a waiting game—one hour then two.

I showered, allowing the water to cleanse and nurture me, with my midwife holding our baby just outside the shower, still attached to her placenta inside of my deep, sacred womb. This was a surreal moment. Time felt warped.

My husband returned home, advising me that our daughters would come home with family friends after their match. Instantly, I remembered back to my first birth. The nurse tugged on the cord, and the placenta came away with intense pain, and I experienced hemorrhaging. Nothing was going to permit this to happen again. The body remembers.

I went into a quiet internal space, now seated on an office chair with wheels, not really the sturdiest kind, and not quite a throne, although I claimed it as one. My energy was spent, and we were in overtime. Holding my babe, I hummed and spoke sweetly to her. "Welcome, sweet little one. I feel honored to be your Mum." My midwife gingerly pushed me on the grey fabric office chair as it wobbled down the hallway to our bedroom; it was in slow motion, an awkward ride!

I was refreshed from the shower and propped up in bed with pillows— wave after wave of exhaustion crashing in. The placenta had not yet come away. I felt a slight panic; we discussed the length of time we could wait before intervention was necessary. There was talk of a hospital visit possibly being needed. It had been about two and a half hours. My mind raced, my body screamed *No!*

I heard voices down the hallway that started coming closer, and our daughters bounded through the door, home from soccer. When I saw the sweet face of our oldest, Harmony, the sight of her automatically expelled the placenta.

I took it as a sign that a circle of healing was complete.

Another shower for me, the bed changed, our baby dressed in clothes, and the placenta wrapped and settled in close proximity. We both rested. Mumma and baby were healthy and content.

August 2003 was mild in Australia—winter. As you can imagine, the placenta is eroding organic matter; in the summer months, this may be less than pleasant. It was not a problem at all. This was a process of allowing and surrendering for us as adults, while it was an honoring one for our daughter. The placenta came away, gently detaching from our babe in a week. We created a family ceremony and buried Lila Persia's placenta in a delightful lotus-shaped planter I purchased.

There is much wisdom, new awareness, and opportunity for both the mother and father in birthing—an opportunity for women to access their power divinely.

"There is a power that comes to women when they give birth.
They don't ask for it, it simply invades them.
Accumulates like clouds on the horizon
and passes through, carrying the child with it."

~Sheryl Feldman

THE TOOL

REJOICE IN YOUR WOMB POWER
FOR LASTING VITALITY AND PLEASURE

This year I turn 60 years young. Much of my healing journey has supported deepening my celebration of all aspects of the feminine and rejoicing in the essence of being a woman. I offer you this tool aligned to your rejoicing.

Our time on the planet is one to be enjoyed. I remind myself often: NOW is the greatest time to expand joy. I feel truly blessed being in a female body. I'm highly attuned to my sensitivities, desires, pleasures, and the divine spark of creation surging through me. From decades leading and being in circles and working with women, I know how hard women can be on themselves.

We must make peace with all aspects of ourselves, bodies, emotions, and our limitations and connect to our innate feminine power. This practice will help guide you to yours. I celebrate you, sweet sister. For your convenience, I have gifted you the recording in my resources.

Create a quiet sanctuary, a place to slow down, to go within, to be. The feminine has a rhythm that is slower than the pace of society. Our cyclical nature shows us this. Truly honor yourself in this way. It is your time.

Turn off distractions. Light a candle. Snuggle a soft shawl or drape a silk scarf around you, a comforting embrace as you turn within.

Sit comfortably with your spine upright and relaxed. Rest back. Our focus is often in the front of our bodies, the position of yearning, grasping, and seeking. Allow yourself to rest back. Focus on your breath and silently say to yourself, drop down, drop down, drop down. Keep focusing on your breath coming in and releasing out, with ease and flow. Slow and gentle. Soften. Scan your body and release any places you're holding tension or stress, bracing, tightening, or resisting. Release it all now. Soften. Sweetly, oh so sweetly, soften.

Close your eyes. Allow your palms to rest against your lower abdomen to connect to your body. With your attention on your breath again, take your awareness to your womb space. Internally travel down to the spaciousness of your feminine. Down. Down. Down.

Rest your awareness here, in your womb. See it as a divine vessel, a sacred bowl. Visualize following its external circumference. See the whole shape of your sacred womb bowl. Your womb space.

Allow yourself to rest fully here. Feel a weightedness, a resting deep down. Resting slightly back. Allow your awareness and consciousness to fill the entire space. Feel the spaciousness. Your womb—your home. Rest.

In the resting, we come to know our power at a new level, reclaiming it fully. Feel yourself connect to the feminine power of creation. Your womb space. This place of nurturing. Pause.

Visualize filling this whole area with golden, liquid nectar. Liquid vitality. Nectar of health. Pleasure. Of sacredness. Wisdom. Empowerment. Of faith. Of wholeness. Delight. Of sweetness. Of strength. Of all the highest qualities of the Feminine. Of the principle of creative energy. Hold the richness and exquisiteness of it all. Pause.

Be at home in this center of power, sweet sister. Pause.

You can rest here daily. Relax, restore and recharge here at any time.

When you feel ready, gently bring your awareness up, up, up from your womb space to your heart space. Fill yourself with gratitude and appreciation for your heart, acknowledging your own self honoring in this precious moment. Pause.

Bring your full awareness back to your body, your seated position, and your breath. Slowly returning. Feeling whole, centered, vibrant, and peaceful.

Continue to use this mediation to help bring more vitality and aliveness, allowing you to savor pleasure at every level.

You can listen to the meditation here:
https://livelifewithwonder.com/collaborative-books

I love original art, it is emotive and a sensory delight I welcome in my life. I have a wall in my office with beautiful original art celebrating the feminine. My soul sister, Jen, calls it my Yoni wall. It is the cover image for my resource for this meditation practice.

As an Art of Feminine Presence Licensed Teacher, watching women deepening their connection to themselves, all their gifts, and the wisdom of their bodies is truly a blessing and a joy. My journey in birthing, motherhood, as a yoga teacher, and a women's coach and facilitator has guided and taught me such richness for womanhood, for which I am truly grateful. Our oldest is now 29, our second daughter is 27, and the youngest is 18, all women of their own empowerment and life direction. I cherish each of them.

I hold a vision and intention for every woman to be empowered within herself, allowing any or all competitiveness to drop away. Sisterhood is sacred. Restoring that is a sacred mission we all can be a part of.

"The wisdom and compassion a woman can intuitively experience in childbirth can make her a source of healing and understanding for other women."

~Stephen Gaskin

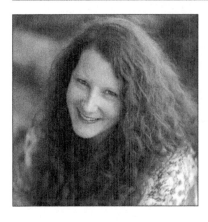

Lulu Trevena is an award-winning author of the stunning hardcover art and poetic prose book, *Soul Blessings*, winning the 2018 Silver Nautilus Book Award. She became a published author after age 55.

She is a Women's Workshop Leader, Quantum Healing Practitioner, Soulful Living Coach, Art of Feminine Presence® Licensed Teacher, speaker, artist, and mother. Lulu is passionate about shifting the societal narrative about women and age. She believes now is the time for the rising consciousness of the planet and for women to live their purpose and passions unabashedly.

She is the creator of the card deck, *Moments of Transformation*, and the hardcover journal, *Epiphany Journal and Playbook*.

Available at: www.livelifewithwonder.com/shop/

Lulu is the Founder and Creatrix of *Live Life with Wonder*.

In 2021 she was lead author of the international Amazon bestseller

Wholehearted Wonder Women 50 Plus: Courage, Confidence & Creativity at Any Age.

In 2020 and 2021, she became a collaborative author in Amazon bestselling books, *The Ultimate Guide to Self-Healing Volume 3; Find Your Voice: Save Your Life; Sacred Medicine: Mystical Practices for Ecstatic Living and The Ultimate Guide to Self-Healing Volume 5.*

You can connect with Lulu at

Website: www.livelifewithwonder.com

Facebook: www.facebook.com/livelifewithwonder

Instagram: www.instagram.com/livelifewithwonder

Email: lulu@livelifewithwonder.com or lulu.trevena@gmail.com

CHAPTER 12

DITCH THE MOM GUILT

EMOTIONAL HEALING THROUGH MOON SCIENCE

Tanya Saunders, MS, LMC

"The easiest way to fail your child simply is to fail yourself."

~Mark Jones

MY STORY

"Bring a picture of your younger self."

My entire body contracted, heat rose quickly from my belly to my chest. *Was I still breathing?* Seconds ago, I was lit up with an inspiring new version of my future. *What the. . .* immediately, images of an insecure girl at awkward school dances with braces, and wiry, tight permed hair flashed in my head. *Was I not specific enough when I asked for natural loose curls? Ugh.*

That request was from the head mentor of a Pause Breathwork Certification I intuitively but impulsively said yes to. At 46, a professionally accomplished wife and mother of three, I'd never encountered such a strange request. *Do they want me to surface my past? Would people think of me differently?*

ONE MONTH LATER

A new day has come.

A new day has come.

I was waiting for a miracle to come.

Everyone told me to be strong.

Hold on, and don't shed a tear.

I was floating above my body and slowly coming back to planet Earth after a meditative breathwork journey. *Is that 'A New Day Has Come' from Celine Dion?*

"Place your hands over your heart, see a younger version of yourself and say, 'I love you, I got you, I love you, I got you.' Thank that young girl for where you are now. Thank that young girl for all that you are now, and when you're ready, roll over to one side, knees to your chest, and wrap yourself in gratitude." *I love you. I got you. Thank you.*

'*Whatever*' would be my ordinary structured mind thinking. In this fetal position, seeing the picture of a little girl that was me and telling her now, "I love you, I got you, thank you," should feel awkward and vulnerable. Yet after the meditative breathwork journey I just experienced, it felt strangely wonderful. *Whoa, this is amazing.*

Lying on the grey yoga mat, I sat up slowly. At that moment, after a 30-minute breathwork journey into my body, my entire nervous system was calm with this overwhelming mind-body-heart-soul connection. *Is this what they mean by oneness?* I noticed I naturally placed both my hands on my heart. I get it now. *This is reparenting the inner child.*

THE INNER CHILD

In popular and analytical psychology, the inner child is the childlike part of a person's personality characterized by playfulness, spontaneity, and creativity. It's how a child feeds their emotional needs. It's what you're born into naturally loving to be and do. As an adult, your inner child is often connected to or closely followed by anger, hurt, and fear attributed to your childhood experiences of being punished, ridiculed, neglected, disregarded, rejected, or abandoned of your emotional needs.

Those emotional needs that you didn't meet metaphorically are now frozen parts that cause adults to feel fragmented, separated, and blocked from wholeness. As an adult, these frozen parts, our inner child needs that are not met, often persist and lead to destructive behaviors. Behaviors include self-sabotage, hostility, anger, depression, or a projection that doesn't serve your highest potential as a woman and as the mother you want to be. These behaviors often leave you with feelings of mom guilt.

PERSONAL DEVELOPMENT

It was two years since I launched what many people term a side hustle. I was a full-time nurse anesthetist for two decades. As an ambitious woman, wife, and mom with a lot of goal-oriented, manifesting, fast-moving masculine energy, I needed to own my time and money as described in my astrological chart.

The launch of a side hustle or an MLM (multi-level marketing) skincare business was also the launch into discovering what makes me special. Meaning, why would someone want to buy from me and not from that other human? *What are my uniqueness and fascination factors?* And so it began. I would consume every podcast, book, course, thought leader, and personality test to learn more about myself. *Am I an enneagram three? Are gifts my love language? I'm a manifestor generator!?* I even launched my own podcast to interview people on their own personal development journey. *My friends were right; I do make a good Barbara Walters.* I'd hear an amazing guest on a podcast, and I was determined to schedule them on my podcast. I craved to know more, go deeper, learn more, and experience and be that best version of me.

THE ASTROLOGY READING

"The sun is your life force, your ego. It's the archetype of Father."

It was my first astrology reading from the book, *Our Cosmic Day* by Leslie Galbraith.

I heard her on a podcast, and my curious nature needed to know more. Immediately I went to her website. "Astrology is a symbolic language for understanding human nature and energetic patterns of behavior. The natal birth chart is a map of your soul's constitution and a guide to track the cycles of experience in your life." *Fascinating.* For the past year, I've been guiding women in mindfulness breathwork circles through the moon cycles. I yearned to learn more myself and to serve my clients.

"You are more than your sun sign, the season when you are born. Humans are multidimensional beings, different constitutions, layers upon layers, elements that direct and influence their personality, their higher self, and their soul." *Ohhh, that's why I always felt guilty about being a weird Cancer.* Memories of shaming and judging myself flooded in.

"Your mom said you were difficult." Words from my husband memorized in my nervous system despite two decades passing. *What a bitch.* I can't believe my mother would say that to my husband when he was respectfully seeking support from my parents before he planned a surprise engagement on a weekend getaway. *What a buzzkill for him. Way to prime my future husband on what to expect in marriage Mother.*

I'm pretty sure he had some idea of what he was committing to. We met when I left the number one ranked nurse anesthesia program in Chicago and transferred to Georgetown for a boy, *which was not my husband.* If that wasn't an indicator of my determined and curious nature, then I'm certain my daily workouts, obsession with healthy habits, and love of fine dining and wine colored his lens of my personality and emotional needs. *My mom just didn't get me.*

My focus returned to the present moment when I was intuitively drawn to Leslie Galbriath's mic drop. "The moon is your emotional needs. The moon is how you give love, how you receive love. It's the archetype of Mother. It's the most important placement to look at in a child's astrological birth chart." *Wow, really?*

WHY THE MOON MATTERS

The Sun and the solar cycle are widely referenced and revered. Seasonal affective disorder (SAD) is commonly understood. Humans are obedient to the sun. The sun dictates the temperature and we adorn accordingly. *Do I really need that coat? Should I wear sunscreen today?*

The moon is not commonly understood with its gravitational pull that predictably controls the ocean's tide, its lunar cycle that is precise and reliable every 29.5 days, the influence it has on a woman's menstrual cycle, and the impact on our water and emotional body. *Did farmers really plant seeds on the New Moons?*

The Moon is symbolic of our emotional needs and our deepest desires. This is important because it is a description of what you loved as a child. How you would give love and how you needed to receive love to feel safe and secure.

This is important because your emotional needs, as described by where the moon was when you were born, can help you identify how to re-parent your inner child. That is because much of what has shaped your emotional temperament now was your experiences before you were conscious of it before the age of seven. The emotional needs you did not meet—those frozen parts that you may not be aware of—still need your love. When you can nurture your inner child, you can remove the blocks known as protectors that keep you from the woman and mother you are born to be.

PROTECTORS

As children, we develop protectors to avoid feeling the pain of our emotional needs we didn't meet. As adults, we don't have awareness around the protectors, and unless we can bring our awareness to it, they'll persist in playing a big role in blocking your potential to expand into the woman and the mother you want to be. When we bring awareness to them by noticing the patterns, we can start to work with them so they're not working against us. *I see you Inner Critic shoulding all over yourself. I should not have eaten that second slice of pizza, I should have this much money in my savings, I should have gone to bed earlier, worked out longer, and not have fed my kids that candy.*

Here are some examples of the most common protectors to fulfill emotional needs:

The Addict

The part of you searching for love, connection, or satisfaction outside of yourself.

The Aggressive

The part that uses fear or aggression outwardly and has an inability to process internally and projects externally.

The Avoider

The part of you that avoids situations you perceive as threatening.

The Comedian

The funny one to break the tension.

The Controller

The part of you that has to shift the external world to feel safe.

The Critic

The part that criticizes what you fear or don't understand.

The Dramatic

The part of you that makes mountains out of molehills.

The Giver

The people pleaser.

The Hyper Aware

The part of you that's always on high alert.

The Manipulator

The part of you that is deceitful and stretches the truth to meet your needs.

The Mistruster

The part of you that is the skeptic.

These protectors may have served you when you were young. However, now as an adult and as a mother, it's time to release and expand not only for the woman you are evolving into, but also for the child you're parenting.

THE TOOL

DETERMINE YOUR NATAL MOON PLACEMENT

1. Go to astro.com.
2. Create a free account.
3. Add New Astro Data.
4. Enter Birth Data Entry.
5. Check "Unknown" for unknown birth time (unless you know, this will give you additional information but is not necessary for this tool).
6. Click on the stored data you just entered
7. Click on "Chart Drawing, Ascendant"
8. Look to the Moon in the yellow box to the left

Astrology is a symbolic language of observation and correlation from over 2,000 years ago. The Moon and the qualities of how it's filtered as described below comes from several of my studies and teachers, but most notably Leslie Galbraith and Debra Silverman. I'm honored and privileged to share the teachings I have invested in, integrated uniquely, and share here as a tool to understand your emotional needs, bring awareness to the emotional needs not met, and ultimately implement practices that can heal your inner child and release your protectors.

Moon in Aries

Your emotional need is to be independent and feel loved by showing courage and bravery. You need a lot of attention and self-assurance. Your inner child needs to win, compete, explore, play sports, and learn new things.

Moon in Taurus

Your emotional need is security. Your inner child is sensitive to your environment and needs comfort, food, and repetition.

Moon in Gemini

You have an emotional need for mental stimulation and to understand everything. Your inner child is curious, talkative, social, and you love to ask questions.

Moon in Cancer

You have an emotional need to be hugged, nurtured, protected, and cared about all the time. Your inner child needs a home that is a nest of tranquility and joy. Mother is very important to you.

Moon in Leo

You have an emotional need to be special, unique, and the center of the universe. Your inner child needs fun and people to celebrate your talents and accomplishments.

Moon in Virgo

You have an emotional need to fix, be organized, and be useful. Your inner child needs to be needed.

Moon in Libra

You have an emotional need for approval, validation, beauty, social, and kind to people. Your inner child needs harmony through love and relationships.

Moon in Scorpio

You have an intense emotional need that is difficult to describe. Your inner child feels deeply and loves control, money, mystery, and deep truth.

Moon in Sagittarius

Your emotional needs are freedom, laughter, and adventure. Your inner child loves to explore, learn, and see the good in everything.

Moon in Capricorn

You have an emotional need for seriousness and responsibility. Your inner child feels loved through tradition, security, and getting good deeds done.

Moon in Aquarius

You have an emotional need for friends and independence. Your inner child looks for collaboration through a unique and unified way of thinking.

Moon in Pisces

You have an emotional need for beauty, storytelling, and daydreaming. Your inner child feels loved through imagination.

GOOD PARENT MESSAGES

The Good Parent Messages used in fields like psychology and counseling, are messages that every child ideally receives to grow up with confidence, emotional health, and self-worth for the skillfulness to grow healthy relationships. They will help you identify your common emotional triggers, patterns, and stories that play out in your life on repeat. After you identify your inner child's needs according to your natal moon, use The Good Parent Messages to deepen your inner child's work by bringing awareness to your insecurities and vulnerabilities that began to form prior to your conscious memory. When you identify your emotional needs in the Moon Sign and discern which Good Parent Messages trigger a "no" in your body, you can rebuild, retro-fit, reparent, and strengthen your unconscious mind by talking to your inner child with these Good Parent messages.

Come into a seated and supportive position. Breathe deeply in through the nose and exhale through the mouth slowly like through a straw for three to five minutes. Be gentle with yourself and go through the list slowly. Notice what feels like a "yes," "no," or "not really" in your body.

- I love you.
- I want you.
- You are special to me.
- I see you and want you.
- It's not what you do but who you are that I love.
- I love you and give you full permission to be different from me.
- I'll take care of you.
- I'll be there for you even when I die.
- You don't have to be alone anymore.
- You can trust me.
- You can trust your inner voice.

- Sometimes I will tell you no, and that's because I love you.
- You don't have to be afraid anymore.
- My love will make you well.
- I accept and cherish your love.

PUTTING IT ALL TOGETHER

Motherhood is a sacred, extraordinary, and soulful experience that you're gifted with. Motherhood is also your greatest teacher. Much of becoming an emotionally healthy mom is an aware woman taking full responsibility for her emotional life. When you can let go of any guilt, blame, or the expectation of others to fill emotional needs for you, you become emotionally free, compassionate, and the highest version of the strong mom you were born to be.

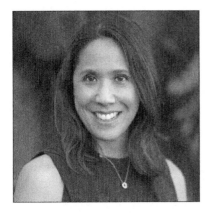

Tanya Saunders is a certified Life Mastery Consultant, Trauma-Informed Pause Breathwork Facilitator, Yoga Psychology Teacher, Astrologer, Author, and Expert Transformation and Manifestation Speaker. She is a survivor of a life-threatening condition, necrotizing fasciitis in 2009, passionate about cultivating a vision-inspired life and helping working women live a harmonious life through breath, positive neuroplasticity, and astrology.

She is the creator of The HEALthy Mind Podcast and HEALthy Mind Coaching, a framework of ancient and modern teachings, practices, and wisdom she has invested in and made her own for strengthening the mind-body-soul connection. Integrating this framework into her 1:1 and group coaching, she has helped women discover their true purpose and manifest work/life harmony through soul alignment.

As a nurse anesthetist for over two decades, Tanya is always learning new ways to bridge science and art to empower the busy, modern woman who desires to manifest a soul-centered life. She lives in Arlington, Virginia, with her husband, three kids, and two dogs.

She has been featured on The Beautiful Grit Podcast with Gwen Dittmar, Everything with Ali Levine Podcast, Keri Faith on Purpose, John Lee Dumas of Entrepreneurs on Fire.

You are one breath and coaching session away from transformation. Are you ready to go on a HEALthy Mind Journey?

Click here: https://bossladybio.com/healthymind

Curious how to connect with Tanya more and where her Virgo Moon loves to serve:

Website: https://www.tanyasaunders.com/

Facebook: https://www.facebook.com/tanya.saunders.520

Instagram: https://instagram.com/tanya_saunders

CHAPTER 13

RELAX, YOU'VE GOT THIS MAMA

FINDING PEACE AND POSITIVITY FOR A STRESS-FREE PREGNANCY AND BIRTH

Lisa Russell, Reflexologist

MY STORY

I was a bundle of nerves and excitable energy as I waited for my husband, James, to come home from work. I was a day late coming on my period, and even though I was like clockwork, I still didn't believe I could be pregnant. It had only been one month of trying, and there was no way we'd miraculously conceived on our first go. We both said we wanted children but were only married for eight months and weren't in a huge rush. I told James, "It could easily take six months, if not longer, so why not stop being careful and see what happens?" But on June 13, 2017 (I remember the date as it would have been my mum's birthday), I saw two blue lines appear on the pregnancy test as clear as day. I frantically marched to the nearest shop and bought three more tests. Yep, definitely pregnant. I was over the moon and couldn't wait to tell James.

"I've got a surprise for you," I blurted out as soon as James came through the door. That afternoon felt like it lasted days. I had been pacing around the front room and was so relieved when I finally heard the key in the lock. I'm also terribly impatient and get overexcited when there is news to share.

"Close your eyes and put your hand out," I continued. I often did this to him after picking up a chocolate bar as a treat. He smiled as if he knew what was coming next, but this time he found himself staring down at a piece of blue and white plastic declaring I was pregnant. Our lives changed forever. His reaction was a bit like mine was initially, a jumble of intense feelings; shock, excitement, fear, and elation. His mouth hung open, and his eyes were wide as they darted back to me and back to the test, followed by manic laughter and a "Yeeeeeessss!" He scooped me up, and we hugged tightly, this new revelation making us feel closer than we'd ever felt before. We popped the cork on the alcohol-free champagne I'd picked up earlier that day and started to get excited about our next chapter.

But as the days and weeks went by, my happiness, every now and then, became overshadowed by anxiety. Intrusive thoughts swirled around in my head like an unwelcome fog.

What if I lose the baby?

I'm terrified of giving birth.

Will I be a good mum?

At this stage, I was quite an anxious person. Having lost my mum at age 15, I was frightened of the worst-case scenario and the possibility of having something else precious taken away from me, especially now that I was on the cusp of becoming a mother myself.

Amidst the anxiety, my heart was swelling with joy, and I knew I would try my very best to be as good a mum as my own had been. I was quite stressed at work too. It's not that I didn't like my job in PR, but I try to put my all into everything I do, and work was no different. But this means I often put myself under a lot of pressure.

I needed an outlet, a coping mechanism to channel my anxiety, replace negative thoughts, and focus on the exciting adventure ahead. This was when I discovered reflexology, and it honestly changed my life.

I started having regular treatments and took up pregnancy yoga. Both of these things allowed me to tune in, slow down, and connect with my baby. Reflexology helped quiet the inner chatter, and I felt so calm, relaxed, and at peace after each session. As my due date approached, I started having treatments more frequently to help to prepare my body and mind for birth.

If you've never had reflexology before, it works by applying gentle pressure to the feet to stimulate natural healing, and it leaves you feeling super relaxed. I was hooked. I remember thinking, *You're growing an actual human being. Now is the time to really invest in your wellbeing.* So I began researching other methods to complement my new desire for all things wellness, and that's when I discovered hypno-birthing.

Hypno-birthing is a method used during pregnancy and birth, which allows you to feel empowered and in control. When I discovered it, I knew it had to be next on my list, and I quickly enrolled in a course. It turned out to be one of the most enlightening classes I've ever taken. It made so much sense to me. It all came back to this basic mantra:

Your body was designed to do this.

Yes, it was! I spammed the walls in my home with brightly-colored post-it notes, which adorned positive affirmations to help me get into the most positive, headstrong mindset I could be in to birth my baby.

The weeks went on, and I continued with my newfound concoction of reflexology, yoga, and hypno-birthing, and by the time 37 weeks rolled around, I was ready. I felt so knowledgeable, in control, and clear on what I needed to do that when my waters broke at 37 weeks plus four days, I put on my hypno-birthing track, and got myself into the zone. I told myself: *You can do this! You'll be meeting your baby very soon.* After six hours, the surges (we don't use the word contraction) became quite intense, so we made our way to the hospital with my hypno-birthing track playing on a loop in the car.

My mind is relaxed, and my body is relaxed.

My mind quiets, my body opens, my baby descends.

I feel confident, I feel safe, I feel secure.

Each surge brings the baby closer to me.

I was at one with my mantras, almost in a meditative-like state, as I soaked up every single word and worked with my breath. I have no idea if James spoke to me at all on that journey. I was so focused. At the hospital, the midwives couldn't believe I was fully dilated. I was taken through to a private room with the most inviting pool I'd ever seen. Any inhibitions I had disappeared at that moment as I threw my clothes to the floor and slid in. I felt the comforting, warm water lapping gently around me, and I felt so safe. After a few chugs on the gas and air and some fantastic encouragement from James and the midwives, my daughter Evelyn (Evie) was born at 8:57, named after my lovely mum.

Since then, I've had another baby, my son George, who entered the world within five minutes of arriving at the hospital. We got off to a slightly dramatic start when my waters broke in the hospital car park, and I barely made it into the delivery suite before his head emerged. But thankfully, it was another quick, positive, and empowering experience, where I was able to use all of my holistic techniques to guide myself through birth. I would do it all again tomorrow. I found birth to be the most primal, amazing experience, and I'm so thankful to my body for doing such a great job at growing and birthing two gorgeous children.

I feel a bit nervous writing this. I know not everyone has a smooth pregnancy or birth experience. I have many clients who've been through really tough times, either trying to conceive or during their pregnancy, and I promise you my intention is not to come across as smug. I know sometimes life throws you a huge, horrible curveball, and some births are particularly difficult. But all I can do is speak from personal experience about how a change in mindset and lifestyle helped me, and I hope it can help you too.

I learned that being confident and kinder to myself, embracing a holistic approach, and believing in myself and my body were instrumental in feeling more in control of my pregnancy and birth. It's something I now try and live by. It's also why I trained as a reflexologist when Evie was nine months old, as I needed to know more about this wonderful therapy that had kick-started my passion for this new way of life.

THE TOOL

Fast forward four years, and as a mum of two, I'm a fully qualified reflexologist specializing in fertility and pregnancy and plan to train as a hypno-birthing instructor later this year. I aim to bring all of the holistic goodness I've learned together, and best serve the lovely pregnant ladies (and expectant dads) who come through my door.

You may be wondering how reflexology helps. The thing about reflexology is that it works on a deeper level than many realize. Although it's primarily about rebalancing the client, removing toxins, and encouraging natural healing, it's also very cleansing both physically and emotionally and sends people into a very relaxed, often dream-like state. This is deeply restorative and helps clients feel rebalanced and function at their optimum, an ideal place to be when you're about to give birth and become a parent.

Clients are told to close their eyes, and we start each treatment with four healing breaths while I stimulate their solar plexus reflex, and they relax their body and let go. We start with the solar plexus as it's our source of personal power and relates to our emotional self. I ask them to connect with the baby and to visualize their perfect birth scenario. Positive visualizations and affirmations can be incredibly powerful. The more you tell yourself something, the more you believe it, and ultimately the more you live by it. Reciting the following statements can make a huge difference:

"I am going to have a smooth pregnancy and a good birth."

"I trust myself and my body."

"Birth is a miraculous and empowering experience."

"My baby knows what to do and the right time to come."

"I will have a calm, serene and positive birth experience."

I repeat these inwardly on behalf of my clients and try to surround them with positive, healing energy. I encourage expectant mums to own their birth experience and help them feel as calm as possible in preparation for the big day. This also helps keep pesky hormones such as cortisol (the stress hormone) from being released during labor which makes us tense up and means we're working against mother nature when trying to birth. Relaxation and a positive mindset will allow your body to relax and your cervix to open and pave the way for producing endorphins—neurotransmitters that act as the body's natural pain killers.

One client came to see me when she was pregnant with her second baby after having a distressing C-section experience with baby number one. We spoke a lot about the importance of removing stress and doing everything possible to stay relaxed and in control, as I believed this would help her the second time around. Each time she visited, we'd talk through other techniques to support her chances of a calm and natural birth, as she was hoping for a VBAC (vaginal birth after caesarean). This included hypno-birthing, of course, as well as acupuncture, walking, and finishing work in plenty of time so she could unwind and mentally prepare for having a baby.

I gave her one of my favorite healing crystals, malachite, a beautiful green gemstone known as the midwife's stone, and I told her, "Keep this close by during the coming weeks." Malachite is believed to resonate with feminine energy, support our intuition, and ease discomfort during birth. I used it myself when my son was born, clenching it tightly in my left palm when my surges began and throughout my labor. I believe it brought me strength and protection.

Back to my client; she did end up having a C-section but had a remarkably positive experience this time around, despite it not being the natural birth she hoped for. She told me, "Through our sessions and from practicing hypno-birthing, I learned it was okay that things didn't go as planned." The difference this time around is that she was in control. In contrast to her first birth, she explained, "I went into the situation feeling well-informed and listened to and I was the one making the decisions about my body and birth." And as a result, she was happily producing colostrum from day one and felt more connected to her new baby compared to her first birth.

"I have learned how important alternative medicine is to the birthing process. I do believe it helped to bring on my labor earlier as hoped along with other things like raspberry leaf tea, eating dates, taking it easy, and no stress," she told me.

I'll tell you more about the benefits of eating dates later on.

Another client of mine had two intense reflexology treatments when she was 39 weeks pregnant, and I used a deep pressure technique around her uterus and ovary reflex points. I used a firm knuckling technique on her pituitary reflex (the pituitary gland secretes oxytocin, the hormone that aids labor and birth). During our second session, she told me she could feel strong sensations in her uterus.

"Just go with it. This is a good sign," I encouraged her. "Your baby will be here soon. You've totally got this."

She started having surges ten minutes after the treatment finished and experienced the serene home birth she longed for with no complications. She believes reflexology helped put her into the relaxed state she needed to be in to kick-start her labor and achieve her ideal birth.

Reflexology can effectively stimulate our parasympathetic nervous system—the state we're in when we feel relaxed, safe, and calm. The exact place we need to be for our body to know it's safe to birth. It's important to say that while reflexology is a great support tool during pregnancy, as reflexologists, we're not wizards, and we can only support what nature intends. But the key is providing a safe space for clients to relax, discussing various lifestyle suggestions to support a healthy pregnancy, and achieving an optimum state physically and emotionally.

Speaking of lifestyle suggestions, I said I'd tell you more about the benefit of eating dates. This is something else I recommend to clients from around 36 weeks after being advised to do this by a nutritionist friend of mine. She explained, "Eating six dates a day in the latter stage of pregnancy helps ripen the cervix and prepare the body for birth." You may never want to eat another date again, but I do believe it helps. Try having them topped with a smear of nut butter, and they are really tasty!

What do I mean by ripening the cervix? Just think of a ripe piece of fruit, let's say a nice, juicy pear. It's soft and tender, and we can easily press it inwards with a thumb or finger. There is no resistance, as opposed to an unripe piece of fruit that is hard and less squashy. A ripe cervix is one more likely to stretch and expand with your baby. I do believe that if you commit to the dates alongside regular massaging of the perineum, the two are a heavenly match to reduce your chances of tearing during birth. Again, I'm not saying this will work for every pregnant lady out there as each experience is different, and babies are, of course, all different sizes. I'm just speaking from my own experience and sharing the techniques I share with my own clients.

This is all part of having a holistic approach, which means looking at your whole self rather than just individual segments. Reflexology is a wonderful therapy, but it can only do so much in isolation. If a client is coming to see me and is highly stressed, for example, treatment will help alleviate the symptoms, but it's also important to identify the root cause and trigger points to support the client. The same is true in pregnancy, which is why I encourage a healthy diet and lifestyle with minimal stress throughout pregnancy and especially in the lead-up to birth.

So if you're expecting a baby or hope to in the future, or even if you're a mum already, just remember to believe in yourself. Talk to yourself in a kind way as if you are talking to a friend. Trust your intuition and don't self-doubt because you've got this, mama.

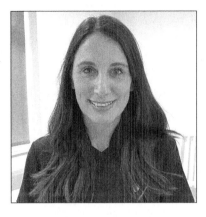

Lisa Russell is a certified reflexologist specializing in pre-conceptual, pregnancy, and post-natal care. She trained at the London School of Reflexology under the guidance of one of the leading reflexologists in the UK, Louise Keet, and has since extended her training to offer facial reflexology and the Zone Face Lift.

Lisa became passionate about reflexology and holistic therapies while pregnant with her first child in 2017 and decided to retrain so she could share her experience and help other expectant mothers and those trying to conceive. Lisa is a huge advocate of hypno-birthing after having two positive birth experiences and using hypno-birthing techniques herself and plans to train as a hypno-birthing instructor later this year.

Lisa is based in Loughton, Essex, in the United Kingdom, and has two children, Evelyn, aged four, and George, aged one. She is on a mission to support expectant mothers and those who long to become mothers as much as possible through her healing techniques, creating a safe space in her treatment room, always offering a listening ear, and providing lots of TLC to her clients.

You can connect with Lisa in the following ways:

www.lisarussellwellbeing.co.uk

Instagram: @LRussreflex

Facebook.com/LRussellreflex

Email: lrussellreflex@gmail.com

CHAPTER 14

MORNINGS MATTER MOST

HAVE THE BEST DAY EVER
WITH THIS ONE SIMPLE PRACTICE

Lisa Lickert

MY STORY

It's early. My pillow feels amazing, and the blankets are snuggly warm on a cold winter morning. I don't know what time it is, but I know I have a crazy day ahead of me. I roll over and check the time. It's an hour before I need to wake up. *Do I get out of bed and start my day, or do I roll back over and try and get another hour of sleep?*

Fast forward to today. The decision is easy. It doesn't even cross my mind to stay in bed, even on a cold winter morning. Who would have thought that the *snooze-loving, let me sleep one more minute, I'm not a morning person, and not going to set that alarm* person would get up early with energy and excitement for each day? Hard to believe? It was for me, too. But after experiencing the power and control created from a simple morning practice on my body, mind, day, experiences, relationships, and life, I'm obsessed with my morning practice and can't wait to share it with you.

I want you to think about a particularly challenging time. It could have been something from five years ago. Maybe it's your current day and the reason you're reading this book. Perhaps you're preparing for a season in your life that is different than those before it, and you're worried. Do you have it pictured in your mind? Now, imagine dramatically and positively impacting the experience with one simple practice. Would you do it? I know I would.

One of my particularly challenging times was about ten years ago. I lost my job as a business executive, where I performed at the top of my industry. My son, who has special needs, was going through a very challenging time. I was the sole income earner for my family. I gained 40 pounds and had frequent migraines. My brother, who was dependent on my care, was battling homelessness, addiction, and suicidal tendencies. I was scared, stressed, overwhelmed, and angry at the world.

I remember crying in my car soon after I lost my job. *What the fuck happened to me? How am I going to support my family? I've let everyone down.* My pity party couldn't last long because I had to walk in the door and look my husband and son in the eye. I was their rock, and I wasn't going to let them down. So, I pulled on my big girl panties and went to work figuring things out.

What did I do to combat the negativity of my situation? I researched, spoke with friends, and sought a better way. Fortunately, I had a few close friends that rallied around me. I fondly remember my friend, Pam. She met me at a function the first week that things came crashing down and asked, "Do you need me to smack you or hug you?" It was a hard question to answer, but it made me laugh the kind of laughter where your whole body is involved. It was great. I chose the hug, and have concluded that everyone needs a Pam in their life.

Finally, a friend recommended a book that introduced me to the morning routine concept. I read it, believed in the concept, and I clung to it like it was my lifeline. In many ways, it *was* my lifeline. I have goosebumps as I think back. I know, without a doubt, my morning practice changed my life. It gave me back my power. I found my spirit once again and the energy that came with loving what I do, who I became, and how I could support my family in every way possible. It was amazing. This new practice paved the way for me to acquire my first business, which included a lucrative deal structure. I lost all the weight and built inner and physical strength. My migraines vanished. Therapies, medical professionals, and programs that matched my son's needs manifested. And my brother secured a home after successfully completing treatment. No joke, and no lie!

There are other stories in my past equally compelling. I've talked with friends, family, colleagues, and even strangers at networking events, and I promise you this, I'm not alone. I bet you've read a book or blog, listened to podcasts, or watched a few YouTube videos on the topic. Are you ready to know how I transformed my life? Keep reading, and I'll share tips, tricks, and recommendations refined over time and unique to busy moms.

THE TOOL

CREATE THE CONTROL YOU CRAVE AND HAVE THE BEST DAY OF YOUR LIFE!

How you wake up each day and your morning routine, or lack thereof, dramatically affects your success in every way imaginable. Scientists have found a correlation between the frequency of brain waves and the body's state. Therefore, what you do, think, and say in the morning sets the tone for the entire day. Controlling your day rather than your day controlling you starts with better focus and being intentional with your morning practice.

When setting a morning practice or routine, there are a few tips I've learned along the way that have set me up for the success I've experienced in my business, family, and life.

TIP #1: DETERMINE YOUR WHY

What's the saying? Your why (why you do something) needs to make you cry. You might think this is a bit much when building a morning routine; however, you'll be tested and tempted to sleep in or skip steps if your why doesn't provoke you to act. What will motivate you to continue if you don't have a purpose for making an effort? As you determine your why, expect to struggle. Dig deep and be specific. For example, if your why involves your children, what exactly do you want for them? Uncover your why, and you'll unlock the first crucial step in getting the life and relationships you crave.

TIP #2: FIND THE TIME

We are crazy busy and typically don't have time for ourselves, so how can you find the time for a morning routine? When people say they don't have the time, what they're really saying is the task or event isn't important enough for them to prioritize it. We can find or create the time if we really want to do something. If you want to watch the latest binge-worthy show on Netflix, you find the time. When you want to shop for a new pair of shoes, you find the time. You want to take a walk after work; you find the time. Right? Finding time goes back to your why. Is there something you do in the morning you can stop doing or switch out? For me, getting up earlier than anyone else, even though I was never a morning person, enables me to complete my routine. This is not an easy task because, in my family, a 5 am start is not uncommon.

TIP #3: KEEP IT SIMPLE

Too much change too fast will cause you to fail, so keep things simple to start. Once you settle into your routine, you'll start feeling great. Managing through tasks is easier, and you'll find a way to carve out more time or add to your routine. For example, if you want to wake up earlier than everyone else in your house, start with 20 or 30 minutes. Don't feel like you need to carve out an hour. Stack activities whenever possible. Have you ever thought about doing calf raises and side lunges when brushing your teeth? Yep, stacking is that simple. Add something simple to an already simple task.

TIP #4: CONSISTENCY IS KEY

A routine takes time to create and master; like a habit, it will form and evolve over time until you get in the groove. Stay focused. You'll experience real results with consistency. Even with great results, you'll still be challenged. We're human. It's not all rainbows and unicorns. Even with the dedication and obsession I have with my morning practice, I can't even count how many times I've faltered. It's normal and expected. So, here are a few ways to help you be consistent and set yourself up for success.

- Post your why bedside so you can see it first thing when you open your eyes each morning.

- Move your alarm across the room. Getting out of bed to hit snooze gives you time to decide if you really should hit snooze. You're already up now. After a while, you won't need your alarm. I haven't set the alarm in years. It's very freeing!

- Create daily checklists outlining your morning routine. Mark off steps as you go. Visual cues help program our brains, and checking off each step gives you a sense of accomplishment.

- Wake up around the same time every day, even on the weekend, this helps you sleep better at night, and it builds a strong desire for sleep throughout the day and helps you fall asleep faster.

TIP #5: WHAT YOU SAY, YOU FEEL

Your thoughts create your experiences. Your words create your reality. Eliminate words or phrases that are self-sabotaging and counterproductive. *I'm so tired. My body aches. I'm not feeling well.* Or the common, *I have to* versus *I get to.* The words you put in your mind or out into the universe can also consume you and override your good intentions. Push the thoughts away and eliminate negative speak. You're a busy mom. You don't have time to deal with negativity.

You're ready to build your morning practice with these tips in mind. If you've tried with limited or no success in the past, that's okay. You should celebrate your desire to focus on yourself and self-care and try again. We learn more from our failures than from our successes, so it's not a lost effort.

Once you have carved out the amount of time you'll devote to your morning practice, think about what you want to include in your routine. Later in this chapter, I share my practice with you and welcome you to use my tried-and-true routine to get started. Common steps found in a morning routine are:

1. Meditation and/or silence. There are free apps to help guide meditation. I like *Insight Timer.* If you choose silence, be purposeful in the time you set aside.

2. Affirmations, Prayer, Gratitude. I recommend you choose what you're most comfortable with and then add as you go. There are free apps and resources to help you create your affirmations, like with meditation. You'll want to start affirmations with "I" or "My." *I choose to be positive. I create happiness and opportunities wherever I go. My life is not a race or competition.* When giving gratitude, list three to five things; this is great to do at bedtime, as well. Consider a gratitude journal, so you can look back during a challenging time to be reminded of all the wonderful things in your life.

3. Visualization and/or scribing. With visualization, you imagine what you want to achieve and mentally rehearse what you'll need to do to achieve it. When scribing, you're documenting your thoughts and insights. You can reflect and detail go-forward opportunities, as well.

4. Reading and/or Audio Learning. This is personal development focused. Learn from experts, mentors, and successful people who've already achieved what you want to achieve. There are thousands of books and podcasts to choose from. Google is your friend here.

5. Exercise. I remember my doctor telling me years ago, *five minutes is better than nothing.* Do whatever you enjoy or try to have some fun with exercise. Hate to run? Take the dog for a walk instead. Need low impact? Maybe a Pilates video in the basement would work. Most don't have time to go to the gym in the morning, but if you do, that's great! Exercise is good for endorphins, good moods, releasing stress, so you have more patience to deal with the hard stuff and the energy to support and take care of your family.

You'll notice I didn't list checking social media, reading emails, or dialing into the news. I know! This may be the hardest habit to break. While many enjoy doing these things first thing in the morning, they're distracting, negative, and stressful. Your morning routine should increase productivity, create a feeling of control, lower your stress, and boost energy.

Find joy and peace in your practice. One way to do this is to create a space for your morning routine other than exercise. Do you have a favorite chair or room? Set up a small table or ottoman for a notebook, journal, inspirational materials, and a coffee or teacup. Think of ways you can make your space special. Let it be known to those who live in your home, the positivity of the experience should be shared, and you may find you will inspire others. Most of the moms I've worked with have never dedicated space to focus on their self-care. You're worth it, so I strongly encourage you to take the time to figure out how you can set something up in your home. For me, it's not my home office, and it's not the kitchen. These areas of our homes are dedicated to activities that focus on other people. I have a favorite spot on our loveseat in the great room. No one is awake but me and my fur baby. He's nestled against me, and my feet are up on the ottoman. It's heaven.

I have several versions of my morning practice. I created variations based on what time my family gets up, the changes in my son's routine and accommodations he needs, my morning meetings, and commute. However, it always includes the five steps, and the changes happen primarily with the amount of time for exercise and personal development. My practice also includes how I wake up and a few tricks I've learned from studying the impact of morning routines. This simple practice I'm sharing with you is the best version and the one I most frequently use.

1. When my eyes are open, I sit up. I have a clock by my bed, so I immediately know if it's close to or the time I need to get up. If it's time to get up and I hesitate for whatever reason, I count backward from five and get out of bed.

2. Drink eight ounces of water. Google this when you get the chance. Drinking water first thing in the morning and right after you wake has incredible benefits; rehydration, cleansing, balancing the lymphatic system, increasing oxygen to your brain, boosting your metabolism, helping aches and pains, helping your skin, and fighting toxins.

3. Brush my teeth. Ridding bacteria that accumulated overnight is the real reason, but brushing my teeth first thing in the morning wakes me up and feels good. I will do the side lunges, and calf raises I mentioned under the Keeping It Simple tip. Sometimes I will stretch when I'm flossing—anything to start moving my body.

4. Dressing in clothes, I can work out in. This is harder than it sounds. Everyone is asleep, I'm trying to be quiet, and I rather put on my comfy sweatpants and not wear a bra. But the moment I don't dress for my workout is the moment I don't do the workout. Even if I

justify putting on my comfy clothes and no bra as something I can wear or not wear and still exercise, it never works. Get dressed. Just do it.

5. Meditation. I select a meditation from my app that's five to ten minutes. I like to lay flat on the floor. Afterward, I stretch a little as I get up and move to my happy place on the loveseat.

6. Give gratitude.

7. Speak five affirmations. I have 25 affirmations pre-written that I choose from. I read them out loud and breathe deeply between each.

8. Pray.

9. Visualize and scribe in my journal.

10. Exercise.

11. Get inspired through audio learning. By this time, my family is waking up, and I'm on duty. So, I will play a podcast as I'm getting ready for the day. I will listen to an audiobook when on the treadmill or walking the dog during my exercise time. I also slip in YouTube videos that I'll listen to or watch when doing laundry, cleaning the kitchen, driving, etc.

12. Make my bed. After I get ready for the day, I always make my bed. Making my bed each morning gives me a sense of accomplishment and a small sense of pride. After a long day, I love walking into my room and seeing the bed made. It makes me smile.

When you first start your practice, watch the time. Time will fly, and you won't finish the routine. Don't get frustrated if it's clunky at first or you can't carve out a full hour. The important thing is to celebrate the time you invest in yourself and your pathway to success. Remember, take control. You have the power to create the control you crave and have the best day ever!

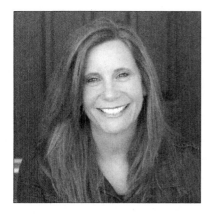

Lisa Lickert has spent the past 22+ years doing crazy awesome things on an adventure to build her best life. She's been fortunate to work in a diverse array of industries and has led, acquired, fought a hostile takeover, sold, integrated, diversified, and built businesses while married to a saint and raising a special needs child. She's a mindset junkie and a wellness goal-getter with a passionate belief in *everything you do matters,* the Butterfly Effect.

Throughout her career/adventure and regardless of the business, Lisa has focused on helping small businesses grow, and people thrive. This is one of the reasons she fell in love with EMI Network in 2012 when she joined as COO and later purchased the company, transforming EMI into a full-service content marketing & creative services firm. Not stopping there, she recently became Partner and CCO of Holland Adhaus.

Her passion for helping and inspiring others to great success has led her to leadership roles with Dress for Success Cincinnati, YWCA, the Goering Center, Redwood, and the Metropolitan Club. Focusing on both the person and the business, Lisa recently launched an owner's forum, with an emphasis on building a business with a purpose, called Cincinnati Catalysts with Success Champion Networking.

Lisa recently launched a passion business coaching moms on their entrepreneurial pathway in a normal serial entrepreneurial fashion. Her programs help moms build successful, scalable businesses so they can take control of their income, their time, and their life.

To connect with Lisa and learn more about her programs, visit https://bit.ly/3jhdIhTFree4Session or https://lisalickert.com

CHAPTER 15

FROM HOT MESS TO HARMONY

USING INTENTION AND INTEGRITY TO GET WHATEVER YOU WANT

Aricka Brazer

MY STORY

Wow. I am a hot mess! I thought. *You're not a hot mess,* I argued back because that's what I do in my head.

You're not that bad. I continue the lie. *No. You are. Stop lying to yourself. It's bad.* The back and forth is nonstop these days.

The dishes are still unwashed, piling higher than ever. The trash is overflowing. Then, I make the stupid mistake of looking at the floor where I see a sticky spot.

What is that spilled all over the floor? It also has hair in it from the dog, so that's been there for a few days. It is sticky!

How did I miss that? Do I need to get my eyes checked? Was it always there?

More thoughts come front and center to my brain. *Great! My kid is crying again. This stupid dog won't stop barking. Doesn't she know that just because the house creaks, it doesn't mean someone is coming in to get us all?*

Well, I chuckle to myself, *let's be honest, maybe that wouldn't be so bad to have something come get us all. That got dark quickly. Who are you, and what have you done with the old Aricka?* I don't even recognize myself anymore.

I was going to take a shower because I am covered in food and boogers, and I haven't slept great since before this sweet child of mine was born-that-I-love-so-much-but-I-really-am-over-all-this-hormone-stuff-because-I-am-about-to-scream! I guess I don't need to shower this hot bod. I can just stay in these clothes another day. No one will notice, right? My boobs are so swollen and droopy. Where are the boobs of my youth? Let's not even discuss this lovely belly sag.

I'm so tired! Didn't I sleep great last night? What time did I go to bed? The baby must have woken up a lot last night.

Wait. That's not true either.

I haven't slept great because I stayed up late watching Outlander again. Then I started watching something else just because I couldn't fall asleep. I don't want my integrity-driven husband, Jonathan, to know how late I stayed up, so I have to wake up early and be cheery. No sleep again, so what are you going to say today, Aricka?

"Hey babe, you look tired. You okay?" My sweet husband asks, concerned.

"Well, we do have a new baby," I say to him quickly.

My brain laughs at myself. I am a comedian. The baby has been sleeping pretty well through the night for a while now. He's eighteen months old, but Jonathan probably won't notice I came to bed late. Little self lies here and there to make me feel better about myself, but how come it doesn't make me feel better?

I wish I was that lady who was like, "Oh my gosh! I forgot to eat!" Unfortunately, I am like, "Hey, I haven't eaten in like five minutes. What can I eat?"

Here is a lovely salad. Um, no, thank you. No green stuff. Where are all my carbs at y'all? It's a carb party over here in my mouth! Not exercising today either so just cross that right off the list. I said I would, but that is not happening. I am way too tired.

"You having a conversation in your head?" Jonathan asks with an odd look on his face.

Where is that look coming from? Why is he making that face? Is he mad? Did I do something wrong?

I look at my phone to find something to change the subject.

Open the calendar. That always works. There's always something to talk about in there. I have nowhere to go, so I don't know why I opened that app.

Wait. I do!

"Shoot! I was supposed to go to that doctor's appointment, but I don't have time to make it, so I guess I'll blow it off again." I try to say this casually because #hotmessexpress over here is supposed to be perfect (in my mind), and I messed up again.

There's that look again from my husband. Is that an eye roll? I know he did not just make that face at me! I feel a tingle roll down my spine as my temper rises.

Hold it together, hold it together, I repeat to myself over and over using my inside voice.

Nope. I am not holding it together this time. I feel my ears get hot.

"Having kids is great because it's the best excuse not to do anything," I say in a snarky tone.

"That is not going to be an excuse forever," Jonathan says.

Why does he always say stuff that's the truth, but I don't want to hear it? Can't he just understand where I am? Nope. That's right. He doesn't get me. I know everything there is to know about him to manage himself. I am his secretary/mother. Awesome. Most of the time, we're good. I am lying. Most of the time, he drives me crazy. Is that his fault or mine?

"How many times can a person walk past the trash and not see its full?" I start to argue.

"The dishes..." he argues back.

"There you go again, trying to make it about me again," I say flatly, cutting him off. I just walk out of the room.

Cool. I am super happy. Not.

Let's move my thoughts to something less about my imperfect marriage.

This missed appointment is a problem. How can I never see people again? I need to see people because I miss people. However, I can't let them see me. I can't let them see the imposter that I am. I have no integrity, feel so gross, and am so sad. If Jonathan tells me one more time that I have negative self-talk, I will explode. Don't you understand I am just a realist!? Okay. That's a lie too. I am so negative and miserable with myself. What can I do? How about another self-help book? Hard pass.

How come all that self-help stuff works for other people, but it never seems to work for me? I start a new year resolution, but by January fourth, it's like reso-what? I'm back to eating the same, staying up late, sleeping in, and freaking miserable. My little string holding it all together is about to snap, and when it does, it's going to be a meltdown city all over everyone and everything around me.

What am I missing? I think sadly.

I am so done.

Maybe your story is a little different, but the feelings are still the same. Miserable with yourself, miserable with other people, can't seem to get it together, frustrated because you want to have it together and you used to kind of have it together, but somehow, it's not anymore. Your relationships aren't that great anymore, and you're pretty sad about how life has turned out.

This is it? I sadly whisper to myself.

When things get overwhelming, I just feel the urge to write, so I sit down when I have a second and write these words.

"I feel like I need a hard reboot. I have so much in my brian that I just feel like I am in a fog."

Wait. I just wrote "brian" instead of brain. What the heck. I do need to go to sleep earlier.

What is it going to take for me to be done enough to make a change? I ask myself quietly.

Then I realized it. It hit me like a ton of bricks. I was like a plane with a passenger list full of promise but no pilot in the cockpit, so I was still sitting on the runway.

I lacked something that a lot of go-getters have. I lacked intention and integrity. Even though I've known about this personal vision tool for years, and knew all the tricks to get more of what I wanted, I only half believed it. I only halfway put into practice the things I learned over the 20-plus self-help books over the years. I didn't have a burning passion for any of the stuff I said I wanted. Most of the time, I felt the stuff that was dealt to me was unfair and totally against me. I didn't have any follow-through and didn't care.

So how was I going to make a change? I was ready. I was done being this hot mess of a woman. I was made for more than this, and I was tired of the life I was living. This couldn't just be it.

I spent some time in thought. I wrote my vision, and then I made a plan for how I would achieve it. I spent a session planning. I needed a hard, fast win. I chose one thing that would help my life the most, and I just did that one thing over and over daily until I mastered it and I achieved what I wrote.

Eventually, with that win every day and feeling like I was living up to my potential there, I added in another thing. I realized I just needed to make the next good choice. When you come to that fork in the road, just choose the best option for you that moves you closer to what you said you wanted.

I fell in love with myself again as I read my vision every day. I realized I deserved what I wrote. I wanted to be that woman. I desired to see her come to life in the fastest way possible, and nothing could stand in the way. Quickly, I realized that she was there all along; I just needed to choose her. It almost seemed serendipitous how things like my schedule, marriage, and mentality shifted to positive when I chose to do the right thing.

THE TOOL

WRITING A PERSONAL VISION

Think about this for a moment. What do you want? Most people do not know what they want. Some have an idea but have never taken the time to write it down or form a solid answer. I know if you would've asked me that years ago, I couldn't have formulated it into even a sentence. I had an idea, but nothing solid.

Most people spend more time planning a vacation than thinking about what they want their life to be like. They say, "I know I want 'X,' but I don't need to write it down." They start to compromise what they want because they're shooting for a moving target.

WHAT IS A VISION?

I've had people ask me, "Is that like having a dream or a goal?" A vision statement is a document that outlines your thought-out purpose and goals. It helps get what you want onto paper (or a device). It helps keep you motivated and focused on the end goal of achieving what you wrote.

Zig Ziglar said, "If you aim for nothing, then you hit it every time."

The vision helps you set boundaries. It helps weed out things that don't go along with your end goal, so you can just say no! You can filter your life through this document. It takes the thought out of these daily gnats that fly around your head and try to influence you to do and be things you don't want.

HOW TO WRITE A VISION

Take a moment to sit down and brainstorm what you want. Some find it easier to dump it all on a page and sort it out. Some like to put together categories and write smaller actionable statements below each category, and some prefer to write it like a story (like a perfect day in your life). Any way you do, it's your way, and that's all good.

Figuring out what's important to you and what you want your life to look like can be challenging. All of us have been influenced, conditioned, and shaped to some degree by those around us and by society as a whole, so it can be hard for us to accurately tell the difference between what we want and what someone else wants for us. Family and friends are a huge factor in shaping who you are, even from a young age. For example, "Everyone in our family always has <insert flaw> or "You are friends with <insert name>, so you will just end up like them too." Those are lies and limiting beliefs you don't have to believe anymore. You're a powerful creator. We are made in the image of God, our creator, so you have that same power to create the life you want. You just have to aim for it.

Once you have brainstormed the idea, I want you to go back through your answers and make sure that they're things you want and not what someone else wants for you. When you look over it, do you feel you're being true to yourself—like the real deep down you you pushed aside all these years? If not, make the changes and reread it. Are the tears coming? Is it hitting a nerve? Keep asking yourself, why do I want this? Or, what is the real feeling behind this want or need?"

Next, write it as if it has already happened in the present tense. Try to avoid phrases like "I want to do X" or "Someday I will..." This part is extremely important because as you read it in the present tense, your brain starts to hear it as an affirmation and starts to believe it. It believes anything your mouth speaks.

Consider your speech for a moment. Does it give life? Is it negative?

There is power in the positive, spoken word. Our words have energy and give life. Leave all traces of negativity out. Don't write what you don't want; write what you do want. The Bible says in Proverbs 18:21, "Life and death are in the power of the tongue." God created this whole world with the words "Let there be," and so it was. Use your words for your good.

There is no right or wrong way. It can be short and simple or long and drawn out. The key is to get it down on paper and start reading it daily. I prefer a one-page document as that makes it easier to read quickly. Pretend like you're five years old, this is Christmas, and there is absolutely nothing off the table. Money and time are taken out of it. Write about the things you stopped dreaming about years ago.

Read it out loud after you've completed it, and you feel like it's the truest, most authentic thing you've ever written. If it's difficult to get through, then you've finished it. There's power in the emotion to change. This is where you find that burning desire.

If you have a spouse or partner, do this exercise separately. Once you both feel it's complete, share it with each other to see where things intersect or if there is something you can help the other achieve. You're on the same team.

HOW DOES THIS VISION COME TO LIFE?

In the Bible, Matthew 7:7-8 says, "Keep on asking, and you will receive what you ask for. Keep on seeking, and you will find. Keep on knocking, and the door will be opened to you. For everyone who asks, receives. Everyone who seeks finds. Everyone who knocks, the door will be opened." This is how I want you to read it and believe it.

Believe that you will receive it, make the best plan that you can, and start taking action. James 2:17 says, "Faith without works is dead." It may not come exactly how you have expected or planned, but that is the serendipity in life. Just be thankful that you have received it when it starts to appear.

TAKING ACTION TODAY

Consider the one thing in your vision that would make the most difference in your life. If you achieved this, it would change your life for the better forever. Take a notecard or small piece of paper and write:

1. The one vision goal. (Front side)

2. The date you want to achieve it by. (Front side)

3. The verses in Matthew 7:7-8. (Back side)

Then make your plan. How can you achieve it step by step? What has to be done monthly? Weekly? Daily? You focus on the daily goal, and it will get you closer to the long-term vision goal. Remember, it's just one good choice at a time.

I did not have enough energy and focus when I started to do more than one thing. I have also found that most of the people I've given this exercise to need to get started on one thing because once that gains traction, they start getting daily drips of the integrity dopamine, and the rest of it comes quickly. Pick the one that will change your life the most and start today.

Use it as a tool to reference if something isn't quite in line with what you say you want. Find safe people to share your vision, don't just share it with everyone. That helps you achieve it faster because they ask you key phrases like, "Is that in your vision?" Place the written vision and the one thing notecard around your home, work, and car. Read it often. The more you read it, the faster you'll achieve it because it's constantly in front of you, guiding you and helping you stay on course.

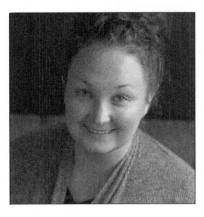

Aricka Brazer is an entrepreneur, and a John Maxwell certified family-relationship coach and life coach. She is currently working on becoming a licensed minister with the United Pentecostal Church International. She coaches alongside her husband, Jonathan, to help lead her clients to live their vision to an intentional, integrity-filled, purpose-driven life. Aricka is passionate about helping others turn their mess into their message.

Her mission is to take others under her wing, as she was taken, and lead them on a journey to become the best version of themselves. She has realized that it can feel like a lonely road at times because of the imperfection we try to hide. She wants people to feel comfortable enough to take off the masks that hide those imperfections and embrace the beauty in their brokenness. From that brokenness comes the healing and change that they desire. It's her desire to live with integrity and intention every day, always striving to do her best and help to heal broken blueprints.

Aricka likes to be at home with her family and her two cats, dog, and iguana in her downtime. She has a passion for hiking and traveling. Branson, MO, is one of her favorite places to be and trout fish with her family. Any place near water is her happy place.

Check out her website for a free resource on the vision exercise worksheet. Connect with her there and through social media:

Website: www.arickabrazer.com

Facebook: https://www.facebook.com/arickafenimore

Facebook Group:
https://www.facebook.com/groups/hotmesstoharmony

Instagram: https://www.Instagram.com/arickabrazer

Instagram: https://www.Instagram.com/hot_mess_to_harmony

CHAPTER 16

HOW TO ACTIVATE YOUR SOUL

THE HEALING CODE FOR COMING HOME TO YOURSELF

Ali Levine

MY STORY

I was spinning on auto-pilot, not knowing what was up or down. I was, for the most part, blissfully unaware of what was going on around me. I was a celebrity stylist. In my ego, I was styling every known celebrity, getting praised, hitting the best-dressed list, hottest parties, soaring new heights in Hollywood, doing whatever celebs needed, stroking egos, taking on their negativity, and wearing other people's baggage with no boundaries for myself. I was a slave to my clients, mentally, emotionally and physically.

I was clueless that I was on autopilot. "Hey Ali, smell the roses. Do you ever take a breath?" My dad questioned. The answer was no. As I became more consumed with my clients and their happiness, I drifted further from mine. I was hitting all the accolades of a stylist, so why was I still unhappy?

Everything had to be a mile a minute. Keep going, spinning, and winning. Externally, I had a fabulous outfit, Louboutin heels, makeup always done, name-worthy clients, New York Times features, VIP invites, red carpets, botox till I couldn't move—you think I'm kidding?

I often thought to myself, *Wow, I really do have it all.* I moved from New York and made it in Los Angeles on my own. I had the top clients I wanted to dress, top publications, flew all over for different projects and more parties—this was life.

In 2017, I was asked to be on camera for different expertise and projects. I went from behind the scenes to front and center! I was asked to be on this Bravo show, and of course, in my ego, I hear, *Bravo, sign me up.* I styled many shows and clients on Bravo. This show was nothing like their regular shows, and instead it was called Stripped, a real docu-series on how you have everything stripped away from you for 21 days and what that does to you. Quickly after signing on the dotted line, I was naked with my husband on camera for the world to see. Talk about vulnerability.

I went from fabulous clothing, jewels, and makeup to *this.* Thank God my husband said he'd do it with me; otherwise, I think I might have passed out on day zero of filming. Thank you, Justin.

Day zero was hard, to say the least. Reality check, you're naked on television, sleeping on toilet paper rolls, and your animals are circling you like something is wrong. Not only are you naked, but you have everything removed from your home. Let's just say there was a lot of tossing and turning and cursing on the first night.

I don't know who was more upset, myself, my husband, or our poor animals that had no idea what happened to their home. The next 21 days were a journey. Every day you got one item back, and you had to explain why you asked for that item. I was convinced on day one that I was getting my phone back and was going to tweet naked, but when it came time, I wanted a dress back. I realized how vulnerable I felt without what I was used to in my everyday life.

I didn't end up getting my phone back until around day four. It was all a blur of high emotions, and 'what the F did I sign up for' moments. As soon as I got my phone back, I checked social media and text messages, and reconnected with the world and my clients—all of it.

My husband got *so* upset with me. "Wow, so glad we're doing this show together. You got your phone back. All is right in the world," he exclaimed.

He was upset because I was no longer talking to him, and I was back in my autopilot zone. This was the beginning of me starting to recognize how not present I was in my life.

One of the producers said, "Why does him saying something like that trigger you so much?" I honestly didn't know why at the moment, and then it dawned on me, he was calling me out for being on autopilot programming all the time. He was calling me out for all the nights I didn't come home before he went to bed and was alone. He was reminding me that I was supposed to be learning on this show, this journey, and since I got my phone back, I wasn't. This was the start to me realizing just how unconscious I was.

The days continued, and we'd have heavy conversations around my career, my husband wanting to have a baby, me not being ready, our life, etc. Halfway through this crazy show, I realized I was facing some pretty dark shadows within myself and how much I'd been hiding behind my styling work and not dealing with much of anything else. I wasn't present in my marriage, and I wasn't present to my friends and family. One of my best friends walked out on lunch with me because I was texting too much.

I wasn't thinking straight. I was mindless. The conversation between my husband and I kept coming up about me becoming a mother, and I kept shutting it down. I convinced myself I wanted nothing to do with it. *I won't be good at this. I don't have the time or space.* I gave myself plenty of reasons to write this idea off. You know the saying, "Man makes plans, God laughs." It was one I grew up around, and my dad always said it. Well, God laughed, and I was pregnant with my first daughter shortly after.

At first, I was scared and unsure, but then this overwhelming happiness came over me, and I never felt so sure even though I had no clue what I was getting into. Boy, did I not have a clue!

Motherhood in itself for any of us—just know it's the most intense ride you'll ever probably go on.

For me, that ride started with a body bounce back that never happened, a water birth dream crushed leading to a transfer to the hospital, to 42 hours later winding up in a C-section and having quite the trauma emotionally, let alone physically. My daughter was here. I was laid up in bed, could barely move, having trouble breastfeeding, my milk had still not dropped, my body was in so much pain, I was staring down at my pretty gruesome cut and laying in bed feeling like, *did this just happen?*

I felt like I was staring at someone else's body and life. I was so happy to meet my baby girl, but I was immediately filled with heavy dark clouds and sadness with the way my birth went and how I felt. This was the start of my postpartum depression.

At the time, I wrote it off as baby blues because that's what most tell you it is. It wasn't, and as I got deeper and deeper and was home, I spiraled further. Between being a new mom, which is hard for all of us, my body was this blob that I couldn't stand. My scar became an ugly obsession. My mind was blank and dark; I had no idea who I was, and I felt like a total fraud. Here I was for years, styling and transforming people with clothing. My motto was: "Confidence is your best accessory," and I didn't have a drop of confidence.

What was wrong with me? I said horrible things to myself in the mirror every day. I would cry some days from sun up to sundown. I was losing it. After weeks of pretending to fix my problem with nail salon visits, massage appointments, and a glass of wine—I did it all, I finally muttered the words to my husband. "I feel like I'm mourning the death of me." Justin's reaction was alarming. He turned and looked at me in bed and said, "What?" I felt like I released something and said, "Yes." I think after saying it all out loud, I realized I needed help. I was diagnosed with pretty severe postpartum depression.

Now what? Get on whatever pills and get back to life? Snap back into the grind?

Something in my soul was telling me it wasn't going to work, and there was more.

I found different therapies to start my healing journey. I remember one of my first sessions was learning about shadow work and cognitive therapy—facing all of my darkness, all the things I hadn't dealt with in my life. There was a lot. Then came time for the next practice and homework I had to do: meditate. "Meditate? I can't sit still for more than two minutes," I told my therapist. She said, "This art of stillness is very important, and you must practice multiple times a day even if you can only last one minute each time."

I remember thinking, *great, I hate meditating, I can't sit still, I pace.* My best friend took me to meditate years ago, and I lasted all of five minutes, until I got my phone and sat on the floor in the back. The reason I share this is because I couldn't meditate to save my soul. I wanted no part of it. Many days and months went by, and I was meditating daily.

I found new happiness in my practice, and when my daughter turned one, and I was able to get dressed and feel beautiful, I thought to myself, *Wow, I am here, I made it. There is light at the end of the dark tunnel.* And there was. Meditation has saved my life in more ways than one. I had a new sense of self, happiness, and who I was. Meditation became my practice.

2020 was a shake, a wake-up—a crash of the ego and a dive into surrender. A new level of trust and letting go. I was pregnant with my second daughter at this time. As the world was spinning and shaking, I did my best to keep myself sane in a not-so-sane world and honor this new life coming in! I was tested all over again. I had to maintain myself, not become crazy depressed at the world and bringing a new baby into it, raise my toddler, and manage my business that was on hold. The list went on.

I thought to myself, *okay, I can spin out because I don't know what the state of the world will be when it comes time to give birth.*

I planned on a VBAC (vaginal birth after cesarean). I just hired my doula and was setting everything up. And there was that word *surrender* in my head again, reminding me it was time to let go and let God. Oof, I did not want to do that. I had all my plans, and they were quickly going out the window. Forget the window. They weren't even near the room.

Every minute the world was changing. There were lockdowns, my mindset was getting worse, and I started to spin, realizing my husband may not be there with me when I gave birth to my baby. Also, I may not have a VBAC due to all the changes in the hospital system; so much was swirling around my mind!

Right then, I remembered how much meditation saved my life with my postpartum depression, and I tapped in. A few minutes into my meditation, my body started to relax. Everything in my body was relaxing. *Ah, yes, this was my happy place.* I remembered what many spiritual advisors and healers told me, the journey outward is inward.

I was back to daily meditation, and back to my routine of coming home to myself. This felt good. This felt right. The more 2020 continued to flip upside down, the further inward I went, back to my meditation with sound frequencies and my new favorite drug, breathwork. Yes, breath can be our drug if we're open to it. Breathwork lets me connect with my energy, life force, and everything.

May rolled around, I fully let go, surrender was in full throttle, and I was going with the flow. My baby girl was testing me harder. Inductions were being pushed on me. Thank God the hospitals had just changed their policy, allowing my husband to be there.

More meditation, breathwork, affirmations, even acupuncture—I tapped in and released all my fears around my VBAC, thoughts of another C-section, and about the actual world.

That Saturday night, we had a dance party with our toddler, pizza, and Hell, I had a glass of wine—all the silliness and fun with my little family of three.

Afterward, I went downstairs for a snack. I felt something. I fell down on my knees and started breathing more into my body, and the tightness increased, so I crawled up the stairs. I crawled into my daughter's room; my body felt weak, but my spirit was getting loud. I crawled onto her rocking chair, balled my eyes out, and spoke my truth about my fears to her little sleeping self, including becoming a mama of two. It felt good. It reminded me that we're not meant to hold emotion. We're meant to release. Wow, was that a release; the contractions got a lot stronger. I drew a bath and texted my doula. She replied, "Get in the bath and get in your zone. I will count your minutes with your contractions for you." I did exactly that. I got into my happy place, put my earbuds in, put my meditation music on, started my breathing, hypnobabies practice, breathwork—the works.

I felt like I was in a portal and already seeing and communicating with my baby girl. I could feel and see her. I never experienced this before. Before I knew it, I was getting louder, and the contractions intensified, and Stacey, my doula, said, "It's baby time. Time to get out of the tub and on your way to the hospital." My husband was sleeping during all of this. He convinced himself she wasn't coming until Monday. Finally, into the truck to the hospital.

I get in my room. I'm already halfway complete. *That was quick.* More breathwork, meditation, movement, and I'm almost complete. *This is going much smoother than I expected, and I'm flowing.* I start pushing, and she gets stuck. All my fears come rushing back immediately. The calm state starts shifting quickly, and I can feel all the emotions building. I hear the words from my doctor, "C-section, if there are more issues." I feel like I'm having an out-of-body experience, and I'm screaming at my body. *I don't have any issues! Okay, breathe, Ali, release, don't tighten up. Don't allow yourself to go backward, trust.* I ask my husband for my earbuds, grab my phone, and put in a fear-releasing meditation playlist; I start listening and pray.

Another minute later, I saw this bright light. It was angelic, and right in front of me. I felt like I was in a sacred portal. I hear my doctor faintly say, "Get ready to push with all you've got." Something came over me and my body and I pushed as I had never used my body in my life. I see a softer pink light in front of me. I feel like I'm slowly coming back to my body, and there she was on my chest. I felt like I was still in another dimension. My husband described it as "postpartum euphoria."

I lay there in gratitude for my body, honoring myself. *Wow, I did it!* I couldn't get the giant smile off my face. I felt so empowered, so strong, I took my power back in so many ways, and achieved my VBAC. As I lay there, I was receiving all the goodness of that moment. I was activated. I was home with myself.

THE TOOL

MEDITATION

GET YOURSELF CENTERED AND GROUNDED

Get comfy. I have a meditation pillow I sit on, a space in my room where I connect to myself and energy. My crystals are around me and my journal next to me, ready to receive any thoughts, ideas, and dreams from my higher self.

I love to listen to Dr. Wayne Dyer and Gabby Bernstein, but the sound frequency is also amazing.

SOUND FREQUENCY

Our cells are always listening. Listening to different frequencies helps our body tune in to what it needs. The modality I use is called SOAAK, where you're soaking in sound frequency, listening to different waves of sound. There are frequencies for mindfulness, anxiety, and body detox. You can go to https://soaak.com/21-day-programs/ali-levine-breathe-in/. If you want to check out SOAAK and SOAK in Sound, as well as experience my breath work, you can use my code: ALI70.

BREATHWORK

My favorite modality. I'm certified in breathwork.

Breathwork is different ways of conscious breathing. It reduces our stress levels, creates openness, and feels more love, gratitude, peace, clarity, etc.

This is the practice: Up, Up, Up, and Away.

Breathe deeply in the nose, three times individually, and then release out through the mouth on away.

Envision you're going up one breathe into the chest, heart chakra, into the throat, throat chakra, into your head, heart chakra, and release. When you release, blow out anything no longer serving you, or you've been holding onto.

You may feel dizzy, vibrating, pulsing, sweating, which is all part of your own magic and your activating of your soul.

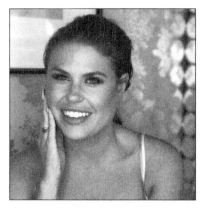

Celebrity stylist and motherhood, fashion and lifestyle expert, and certified breathwork specialist. **Ali Levine** believes that no matter where you roam, from the laundry room to the red carpet, authenticity is your superpower, and "confidence is your best accessory." Raised in the high-velocity fashion culture of NY, a natural gift for style led Levine to opportunities working with corporate design. A transition to television/film took her to Hollywood, where she founded the Ali Levine Design Headquarters, quickly establishing herself as LA's "it" girl of celebrity styling with a star-studded portfolio.

After the arrival of her first child, daughter Amelia Rei, Levine wholeheartedly embraced the role of mompreneur and mommy influencer. She is now a mama of two and shares her real raw truth of motherhood. She is a sought-after motherhood style/lifestyle expert covered by Forbes, The Wall Street Journal, and NY Times, and she has been named on the top 40 fashion blogs. On the "Everything with Ali Levine" podcast, the style maven and mompreneur, Ali delivers a real, raw look at her own motherhood journey amid the treasures she's uncovered in the universal search for authenticity, spiritual wholeness, and happiness.

True life inspirational interviews on the 5-star rated "Everything with Ali Levine" podcast on iTunes. Ali is releasing her spirituality podcast on 2/22/22, called Awakening With Ali, all about her own spiritual journey and awakening and activating herself.

When Ali's not busy transforming others, sharing her real and raw self, using her voice to empower others to live their best authentic lives, you can catch Ali playing outside with her daughters, having a date night at home by the fire with her husband, trying on outfits in her closet usually with her little fashionistas, dancing around, laughing, taking walks, eating something chocolate and diving deeper into her practices.

Connect with her on the following sites:

Website www.alilevine.com

www.facebook.com/Alilevinedesign

Twitter: www.twitter.com/Alilevinedesign

Instagram: www.instagram.com/Alilevinedesign

LinkedIn: https://www.linkedin.com/in/alilevinedesign/

CHAPTER 17

THE WAY OF THE WARRIOR MAMA

PRACTICING THE WISDOM OF FEARLESS SELF-CARE

Laura McKinnon, ERYT

MY STORY

It was the day of my third doctor's appointment with the pregnancy of our daughter, and I was full of worry. The pregnancy came 15 months after our second child died unexpectedly at birth and presented a myriad of complex emotions.

Waking that morning, but before my eyes even opened, I felt a hollow sensation in my stomach and tightness in my chest, the all too familiar sense of dread. Panic began to take hold, an unwelcome foreign invader seizing my body and flooding my senses with fear. My mind finally caught up with what was happening as I tuned into my shallow breath.

My first two doctor appointments went well, so I was incredibly disappointed to be having this reaction, especially after the pep-talk I gave to myself the night before. Knowing that worry may try to work its way in, as I drifted off to sleep, I repeated to myself, *Laura, you know that everything will be okay. You can't control what's going to happen, so let go and trust God. You're in good hands, and no matter the outcome, you will be supported, and you will get through it. Breath. Relax. You can do this.*

The moment I awoke, my body and emotions clearly hadn't gotten the memo, or if they had, they were no match for any intellectual reasoning. Emotions overpowered me with such force that I did what I could only do at that moment, bury it and push it away. I didn't have time to deal with panic and worry, and perhaps more honestly, I didn't *want* to deal with it. I desperately wanted to run and hide from my fear or shake it off like a dog just out of a bath. *How dare panic arrive unannounced, not checking in with me first?* Ignoring the unease and determined to move through my day as normally as I could, I pulled myself out of bed.

My morning was anything but normal. The more I tried to push worrying thoughts away, pretending everything was just fine, the louder my fear became. I tried sinking my attention and energy into the tasks that needed to be done, but fear had its grip, and it wasn't letting go. By the time I arrived at my appointment, I was on the edge of a full-blown panic attack. My forced smile in an attempt to cover my emotions felt like a dam about to break, causing catastrophic destruction. Swallowing back tears and wanting to scream, my body felt like it would crumble.

Pull it together, Laura. You can't fall apart in front of all these people. You've come too far to let this one appointment take you under. I took a deep breath and waited for what felt like an eternity to be called. I wanted to both delay and rush the appointment at the same time. *For heaven's sake, I just want this to be over!*

Finally, the nurse brought me to the exam room to take my vitals and ask the usual questions, only I barely heard what she said, and don't remember how I replied. It was like I was stuck in a vacuum, unable to hear and see anything around me. I was consumed with trying to breathe. Minutes later, my doctor walked in. His soft but commanding and loving presence started to take the edge off until I noticed another man directly behind him. "Laura," Dr. Chandler said, "This is Dr. Howard. He's training with me today. Is it okay that he's here with us?"

"Yes, Dr. Chandler," I lied as my mind screamed, *No! I don't know you, and I don't want you to see that I'm falling apart!"* I somehow managed to gulp back my emotions even though I was desperate to let them out. My doctor gave Dr. Howard the lead, handing him the fetal doppler as I was instructed to lay back on the table. "Time to listen to baby's heartbeat!" He announced. My throat tightened as breath left my body. Instantly I understood that it was this specific moment I'd been dreading. *What if there's no heartbeat? What will I do? I can't go through losing a baby again!*

Dr. Howard started moving the doppler around my belly. Nothing. He moved it around again—still nothing. Time seemed to be standing still as he lifted his hand to move the doppler again. Sensing my angst, Dr. Chandler stepped in and, taking the doppler, said, "Here, let me. These are tricky sometimes."

Ba bump, ba bump, ba bump, I heard as Dr. Chandler set the doppler on a different area of my belly. An audible cry released from my throat as tears of relief streamed down my face. I would have instantly crumpled to the floor if I'd been standing. The intense and agonizing emotions gripping me all morning immediately emptied.

Later, when I arrived home, I reflected on what I experienced. I saw the fear that taunted me all morning long. I could taste its residue in the back of my throat and feel it in my body. When I awoke that morning, I refused to address it. I refused to name it. I attempted to ignore it, and I suppose because ultimately, I knew there was *nothing* I could do to ensure my baby had a heartbeat. It was out of my control, and that alone terrified me.

I spent the rest of my day unraveling what the experience did to both my mind and body. It wasn't pleasant, and it took me time to recover. I remember thinking, *Is this what I'll have to endure for the next 25 weeks?* But I knew I couldn't go there. I understood that worrying over the next 25 weeks would not only cause mental and emotional agony but keep me from being present, moments I could never get back. I decided to settle with knowing that fear would come. I may not see it coming, but I couldn't ignore it. I needed to face it and address it. I knew the *only* way to overcome fear was to see it and move *through* it.

From that day on, I started calling myself *Warrior Mama*. I leaned into everything that connotes a warrior and worked to embody it. There was no room to pretend or become a warrior only part-time. It was all or nothing because that's how I deemed a warrior to be. A true warrior is a warrior by nature, not just some role to play. For me, becoming a warrior mama was out of necessity to keep fear at bay. I wanted to feel empowered and strong for myself and my baby. It wasn't long after beginning my journey that I understood being a warrior mama was a way of living.

As mothers, we constantly navigate through the seemingly impossible with unsurmountable expectations. There are moments when motherhood may feel natural and effortless, but it often drains us completely. We're expected to pull off victories like an Olympic gymnast, perform miracles like a revered saint, settle quarrels like a wise guru, and organize chaos like the CEO of a Fortune 500 company, *all at the same time!* It seems assumed that mothers are unending sources of energy and knowledge. But where is our training? Don't get me wrong, mothers *are* completely badass and *can* make possible the impossible, but in my journey, I had a revelation of what seems to be missing most in motherhood—seeing ourselves as warriors and taking care of ourselves as one.

The word warrior is defined as "person who fights in battles" and "known for having courage or skill." Mothers certainly fit this. Do we not engage in battles on a daily with our children? I don't know of any other occupation that demands more than being a mother. Being a mom is *all day*, 24/7, and fighting battles is just one of our many duties.

So how do we become a warrior mama instead of an exhausted, burned-out one? It starts with understanding not what a warrior *does* but what they *are* and *how* they come to be.

There is a difference between acting as a warrior and *being* one. If *being* a warrior is who you are, your warrior-ness doesn't end when you step off the battlefield. It's in *everything* you do. When I looked up *"What makes someone a warrior?"* I found:

"A warrior is someone who understands their needs and is fearless in telling others what they are, even at the risk of being vulnerable."

"A warrior is fearless in living."

"A warrior knows their gifts and develops them throughout their life."

"A warrior knows suffering."

Whoa! Can I get an, "Amen?"

I confess I've never been to combat training to prepare for warfare, but I surmise it's quite extensive. This training would include tools to optimize the physical body's health, increase stamina, endurance, and clarity, develop the strategic ability to be one step ahead, how to move with force and not against it, and above all, to carry grace and wisdom in the heart.

Mothers may be gifted with intuitive abilities we never knew possible, but it's how we use and care for them that matter most. Being a mom doesn't have to be an overwhelming identity that sucks away our life force. It's completely possible to refine our skills and walk the path of motherhood with stealth and grace, without losing ourselves and our minds in the process. *Hence, The Way of the Warrior Mama.*

Warriors prepare for what they know is coming *and* for the unexpected. Battles often arrive suddenly and unexpectedly. They don't care if we're on zero hours of sleep or haven't had our coffee. There will always be times we must go at a moment's notice, but if we prioritize *ourselves* through practices that support our well-being, we build stamina and readiness for them. If we train like the warrior mamas we are, we become better prepared and able to use our acquired tools.

This is the wisdom that comes with the Way of the Warrior Mama, first seeing and acknowledging our inherent greatness, then having the burning desire to support our greatness. We must know our needs, express them, and nurture them. We must recognize our innate gifts, celebrate and develop them, and learn how to use our suffering to empower ourselves. This is what allows for fearless living. Rooted deep in our body and heart is the innate wisdom of the warrior mama who can conquer everything that is handed to her.

Self-care is non-negotiable. It isn't a luxury or nice thing to do when we have time. It's an absolute necessity. We must fill our cup before showing up for ourselves and others. Self-care feeds empowerment, the recognition of our inherent strength and wisdom. When we commit to ourselves, it connects us to our own worthiness, and when we value ourselves, we're no longer willing to sacrifice our wellness. Self-care doesn't have to be complicated or take a lot of time, but it's important to be consistent. Consistency is what builds stamina and supports readiness. The Way of the Warrior Mama cannot be lived haphazardly. You must first see yourself as the warrior you are to begin walking the path.

THE TOOL

A DAILY SELF-CARE PRACTICE TO AWAKEN AND STRENGTHEN YOUR INNER WARRIOR

I begin my day with quiet time dedicated to prayer, meditation, and simple movement every morning. This routine wakes up my body, creates clarity in my mind, and sets the tone for the rest of my day. It takes ten minutes or less. You can add in other practices/movements if you have more time but beginning with what is manageable is key for consistency. You can do it any time of day, but I recommend it be the first thing you do when you awake, as it can set a powerful tone for your entire day. The Way of the Warrior Mama calls for your daily practice to be a ritual, an act done with intention and sacred devotion.

Begin by lighting a candle. Look at the flame, take note of its light and let it remind you of the light and fire within you. One option here is to add incense or essential oils in a diffuser as scents can enhance/support your mood.

Offer a prayer of gratitude, calling for support to be the best version of you, seeing the grace, goodness, and beauty in all things.

Sit comfortably (on the floor with a cushion or a chair) to ground yourself. Feel your sit bones and let them anchor you into the earth. Sit tall, lengthening the spine from your tail up through the crown of your head.

Close your eyes and connect with your breath. Notice the quality of your breath, the length of the inhale and exhale. Consciously begin to even out your breath, let the rhythm become smooth. Keeping an even rhythm, gradually expand your breath to become deeper and slower. Stay with your breath for several moments. If you feel anxious, let your exhale become longer than your inhale.

Visualize healing energy moving up from the bottom of your feet into your pelvis on your inhale and pouring down through the crown of your head, filling your torso on your exhale.

When ready, gently open your eyes. From the shoulders, rotate your arms outward, inhale, lift them overhead, join the palms together and lower down in front of your heart on the exhale. Repeat a few more times.

Place your right hand on the floor or chair. Inhale the left arm up and side bend to the right. Keeping both sit bones anchored, allow the length to originate from your waistline and extend up and out through your top arm. Repeat to the other side.

Take the right hand behind you, the left hand to the outer right leg. Inhale, lengthen the spine, exhale twist to the right. Stay for several breaths, inhaling for space, exhaling to deepen the twist. Feel the rotation in your upper back, allowing it to release tension. Gently release on an exhale and repeat to the other side.

Take several rounds of cat/cow to move energy and support suppleness of the spine (you can do this seated or on all fours). Inhale, tilt the pelvis forward, creating a slight arch in the upper back as you lift the heart upward. Exhale, tilt the pelvis back, drawing the navel towards the spine, slightly rounding the upper back, chin towards the chest. Do five rounds.

Move into extended child's pose, taking knees wider than hips and drawing feet together. Hinge at your hip folding forward, walking the hands and arms out in front of you to lengthen the spine. Rest the forehead onto the ground or on height (such as a folded blanket) to support your neck. Keep hands shoulder-width apart, press the palms down and forward and draw the outer hips back. If using a chair: stand facing the chair taking your hands to the edge of the seat on either side. Walk your feet and legs back, folding at your hip until feet are hip-width apart under your hips, torso halfway down. Press your hands gently into the chair as you draw your outer hips back to lengthen the spine.

Rise to standing. Balance into the four corners of your feet and press the feet down to strengthen and engage the legs. Lift up through the arches of the feet, drawing energy up the legs, supporting the tone and lift of the lower belly in towards the spine. Lift your collarbones, extend the spine through your crown, and reach your fingers towards the floor. Tune into the strength and stability this posture (mountain pose) offers.

Find a heavy, sturdy piece of furniture slightly higher than your hips. Stand two feet away in front of the object, legs slighter wider than your hips, toes turned out slightly. Place your hands onto the edge of the object to hold firmly. Use the leverage to support bending your knees, lowering down into a squat (to lessen the bend in the knees, you can use a rolled blanket behind the back of the knees and/or don't come all the way down into the squat). Let the tail lengthen towards the floor as you lift through the heart. This pose releases the lower back, tones and massages the organs in the belly. Connect to your power source, the womb wisdom in which we create and birth life. Allow this womb wisdom to flow into your heart as it rises, supporting you as you awaken your inner warrior.

Come back to standing, join palms together in front of the heart, say to yourself, "I am a warrior mama. Let it be, and so it is."

Additional Warrior Mama tips:

- Ask for help when you need it.
- Learn what feeds your soul and do more of it.
- Spend time in nature, with ample sunshine and fresh air.
- Sing your heart out, dance like no one is watching.
- Find your internal rhythm, commit to choosing things that support it.
- Journal when your mind is running wild. Let your thoughts release as they fly onto paper.
- Take a warm bath or shower with your favorite scented soap.
- Read a juicy novel.
- Let go of guilt—*all* of it for true warriors live in the presence and peace of their own hearts and never apologize for it.

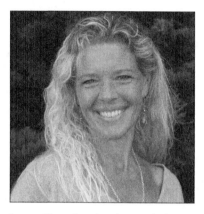

Laura McKinnon is a yoga teacher, writer, and mother. With her love of yoga and joy for life, she encourages students to meet themselves where they are, cultivating self-love and compassion to ignite the bright light within. Woven into her classes is the practical wisdom of bringing yoga into daily life. Her certification in Grief Yoga® helps her assist others in moving through grief, transforming sorrow, and reconnecting to love. She also leads workshops and teacher training at her yoga studio in Carmel, CA. As a lover of nature, you will find her most often outdoors in two of her favorite places, the ocean, and forest. She resides in Seaside with her husband, three children (two earth angels and one heaven sent), two cats, and a dog.

Connect with Laura on the following sites:

Website: laurasrainbo.com

Facebook: https://Facebook.com/LauraMcKinnon

CHAPTER 18

THE YEAR OF NEAR DYING

SURVIVING THE PREDICTED DEATH OF A CHILD

Pamela J. Pine, Ph.D., MPH, MAIA

MY STORY

Dropping my daughter Lisa off on her first day of college in September of 2012, I could see she was a bit scared, not atypical for a young person just off to college. It can be a somewhat iffy time emotionally. She was a sensitive kid, and being on one's own can be trying when one is like that. When she called the next day, I sensed panic in her voice. "I'm not happy, Mom. I'm worried about my classes and about getting along with my roommate." More calls from Lisa in the following days and weeks indicated loneliness and mild depression. I was concerned but not overly. She needed to adjust. Lisa went to see a counselor for guidance who prescribed an anti-depressant. The combination worked well. Lisa thrived, made good friends, got involved in activities, and did well in her classes. And her blond hair, gray-green eyes, delicate features, and long, shapely form helped her get attention from everyone, including the boys.

Upon graduation four years later, Lisa took a paid internship in upstate New York, helping newly arrived refugees enroll in school and fill out forms while introducing them to American ways and habits. She loved the people and the intercultural experiences, and everyone loved her. During a visit to a farmer's market when I visited, Lisa introduced me to an Afghan man who sold household wears. He had nothing but compliments. "Your daughter is one in a million. She is kind and helpful and thoughtful and smart. We love her." I felt proud. I felt like I had done a good job!

Everything was going well until it didn't.

A year later, in the summer of 2017, Lisa and her closest friends from college decided to live together in Arizona and hang out for a while. This was when things began to unravel. The heat was oppressive, and painting houses and working with a local charity was unfulfilling. An owner of a business she was painting for made unwanted romantic advances. When she did not reciprocate, he fired her. At the same time, her tight friendships became strained over living conditions, boyfriends, and communication problems.

When she started to have additional issues with depression, Lisa took it upon herself to lower the dose of the anti-depressant she was taking, deciding the meds were harmful. She called home more often. "Mom, I'm really depressed. I don't know what to do." We talked through it, what was wrong, and what she could do. Lisa concluded most of her problems were related to her medications and so decided to go cold turkey, with no psychiatric check-in. It was a bad decision, and I told her so. Her state of mind further deteriorated.

She decided it was best to leave Arizona. In the fall of 2018, she returned to upstate New York, where she'd been so happy. But she only got worse and felt lost. She was embarrassed amongst friends who knew her as a different and happier person. A refugee friend, just being straightforward, asked, "What happened to you?" This made her cry, and it made me nervous.

Desperate, she hiked with a formal program in the mountains in Colorado to address her depression and visited cousins in California, only to return home no better and at her wit's end over what to do next. She refused the possibility of all medications, thinking they were dangerous and useless. No exceptions. Social media became a stumbling block to her healing. She found countless articles on how the medication did more harm than good. I disagreed, but I was fighting a losing battle. I began to feel like I was living life either in slow motion or in fast forward.

We went to see another psychiatrist in the late fall of 2018. He recommended doubling the dose of a medication, and Lisa expressed concerns regarding its addictive properties. The doctor dismissed her concerns. "Well, it's better than feeling like this!" he said.

After we continued expressing doubts about his recommendation, he suggested a procedure called Transcranial Magnetic Stimulation (TMS), a treatment whereby a device is placed on the head and beams magnetic forces to the specific part of the brain implicated for depression. We were told it could help people who don't respond well to medication. He said there was no downside. "It won't hurt you if it doesn't work." Lisa and I were dubious.

We got a second opinion; there were no possible negative consequences. However, they did not mention that undergoing TMS soon after coming off psychiatric meds could be harmful (a warning we eventually discovered while researching the equipment's manufacturer).

We decided to do the procedure. It was a mistake.

After her first session, she could barely get out of the car after arriving home, and I had to help her into the house, holding her under her arm. We reported this to the clinic, but it fell on deaf ears, and staff discounted it as a possible side effect. After the third session, Lisa came home out of control and banged her head against the wall. She called the TMS office again, demanding that the staff be more forthcoming and responsive about what was going on. However, they insisted that sometimes there was a "dip" when doing TMS. "Some patients report worsening of symptoms for a time before they get better," the technician said. They encouraged her to continue the treatment.

In these few weeks since starting TMS, Lisa's behavior and personality were radically changing. She would not talk to friends and did not go out because of the anxiety she experienced in meeting anyone, even people she knew.

We were both now beside ourselves with what to do next. Concerns expressed in calls to the office went unanswered or dismissed. Lisa developed tachycardia, an unusually high heartbeat. Pills were dispensed to calm her down, and the office suggested additional treatments. We did not know what to do. We struggled for a long time with her severe depression, then anxiety, then Lisa's rage and insecurity.

With a final treatment in late December, Lisa was left more depressed, unable to speak, and less mobile. My outrage kicked in, and I demanded to talk to the doctor. We went in. The psychiatrist dismissed her and said her symptoms could not have been caused by TMS. We now not only had questions about the procedure; we questioned the doctor's competency.

Lisa went to see a neurologist. After she started crying over concerns about her health, he dismissed her. "What are you doing here? I can't help you. Please leave."

Over the next four months, she suffered from constant anxiety, panic attacks, facial tightness, nausea, headaches, dizziness, heart palpitations, and fatigue. She was not getting better.

In the late winter, I took Lisa to a nearby psychiatric inpatient hospital with an excellent reputation. They gave her a new medication every day with no results. At one meeting, the psychiatrist leaned over the desk and aggressively asked, "Well, if you don't want to take the meds we've offered, what meds *do* you want to try?" At the hospital, a patient overheard a nurse practitioner say Lisa was the hospital cry baby. The hospital released her a week later. We felt lost.

Over the next several months, Lisa saw multiple general practitioners, neurologists, and other physicians. While looking at other treatments for depression, she tried several outpatient clinics, besides calling numerous researchers, experts, and TMS practitioners. In her research, she discovered studies showed a potentially negative relationship between TMS, the autonomic nervous system and heart rate, and the possibility of severe headaches after TMS treatments. One study underscored possible increased anxiety. Our utter confusion, dismay, and now fury, continued.

One morning in early September 2020, her father came over to go for a walk with Lisa but couldn't wake her. He came to tell me. I ran upstairs, moved her limp body to the floor, administered cardiopulmonary resuscitation (CPR), and screamed to her father to call 911. We had no idea what had happened to her. There were no bottles or vials in the room. I had been controlling her medications. I had only given her one tranquilizer the night before because of her high level of anxiety. Still, we assumed the worst, that she had tried somehow to harm herself with some type of medication.

The EMTs arrived and continued CPR, hooked her up with oxygen, paddled her, and took her to the hospital. At 2 am, the hospital called me. Lisa was very sick, they said. They flew her to a hospital where she could receive a higher level of care. I arrived as they put her on breathing support and inserted a feeding tube. Her kidneys and liver were shutting down. They administered medications and hooked her up to kidney dialysis. I was in disbelief and overwhelmed with grief.

The next day, the information came at me as if in a dream. The doctors told me Lisa had suffered a cardiac arrest, which limited the amount of oxygen to her brain, causing extensive brain damage, affecting motor coordination, short-term memory, and loss of her sight. The doctors did not think she would live. If she did survive, they said, she would need both a liver and a kidney transplant. And she would probably not be able to walk again, given the extent of the damage to the cerebellum, which helps with coordination and movement, and the damage to support short-term brain functions. So, even if she took a step, she would not be able to retain the learning of how to walk. If she lived, she would likely be a blind quadriplegic with little or no life fulfillment. The only news that could have been worse was that she had died.

I sat in a meeting with her father and the primary staff involved with her care on a Zoom screen. The Palliative Care Department at the hospital concluded she would not have much of a life if she survived. They said I had only a small window to decide. If they removed the breathing and feeding tube, she would die. As a single mother, it was up to me to decide what would happen to my baby. I asked if they were certain Lisa would unlikely recover and reengage in life. They said, "It's pretty darn sure she wouldn't." I asked about brain function and young people's recoveries I read about. The hospital staff reiterated it was unlikely she would recover. I looked at the Zoom screen and more than said, moaned, "We are going to lose her," and broke down crying, "I can't do this!"

I asked to speak with the head neurologist of the eight-member team of doctors and nurses, who gave a glimmer of hope. "You don't need to make a decision now. The fact is, this is the brain, the last frontier, and we simply don't know what is going to happen. She is young, and she has that in her favor," he said. I decided to forge on. Coming home, sitting on the back deck of my house on an unusually sunny and warm September day, I called a friend. "I have no idea if I'm doing the right thing," I told her.

The next day when I arrived at the hospital, Lisa was sleeping. I put my hands and arms across the guardrails and my head on them and wept.

I'm not a religious person but I *am* spiritual. "Please keep my daughter in your thoughts," I wrote to my friends. I hardly knew what to say. I provided no details, partly out of privacy but partly because I didn't want a surge of "Oh my God" and did not want to explain things over and over to people. "Please focus on hope and healing," I pleaded. Many, many people did.

I went to the hospital every day, staying all day. I brought headphones and played her favorite music while she was unconscious. After about a week, Lisa gained consciousness and began singing to the music coming out of the headphones. I brought scented oils for her to smell, and she chose her favorite for me to put on her. I brought photos of family and friends for her to possibly see.

For two weeks, Lisa could not move an arm, leg, foot, toe, finger, or a single part of her body except her neck and head. One night, she called me. I did not hear the phone ring, so she left a devastating message. "Mom, I can't move. Why can't I move?" she said pitifully. She did not know where she was from day to day and could not remember hospital staff, much less their names. Tony, a nurse with a wonderful sense of humor and demeanor, always came in the room asking, with a smile, "What's my name?" which led to his new name, "Tony What's My Name." He has become a family friend.

After two weeks, Lisa regained her sight. Then, she slowly began moving her fingers, arms, toes, and legs, followed by remembering all her friends' names when I showed her photos of them. She continued singing along to her favorite music. Her kidneys and liver healed. After a month, she still could not walk or use the bathroom alone, and she couldn't concentrate enough to read and remember. Still, she was making progress.

Lisa's father and I spent four hours on Zoom with the staff of a rehab facility with a reputation of being one of the world's best, talking about brain injuries, their consequences, and Lisa's situation. They smiled and nodded—they understood. "We can help her," they said, and a few days later sent a private jet to pick Lisa and me up and transport us to the rehab center. Finally, there was hope.

Within five days of arriving at the rehab center, Lisa was walking somewhat unsteadily and with some assistance, but walking. I took a video of this—Lisa is crying, and I am saying: "Lisa, I am flipped out; I am floored. Oh my god, Lisa." We had a future.

She stayed five weeks, taking part in physical, occupational, psychological, music, and art therapies. I spent many sleepless nights on the cot next to her bed. They put her back on anti-depressants and worked with her hours every day. When she was discharged, her 5'6" frame weighed 95 pounds, but she left the building walking with braces on her lower legs and had full use of her arms, hands, and fingers. She continued having some short-term memory problems, not remembering conversations from minute to minute, but ultimately, she remembered where she was and why. I could not have been more grateful to those caring people at the rehab center.

We returned home the second week of November 2020, where she continued cognitive, physical, and mental health therapies.

A year later, Lisa had recovered about 98 percent of her physical abilities and walked without braces and with hardly a hint of anything having been wrong. Her abnormal heart rate is gone, and she has discontinued most of her medications. Although she doesn't remember everything, her short-term memory is back for all practical purposes. She remembers where she is and was, most of what happened, and has full and complex conversations. She has gained 25 pounds and is almost back to her normal weight. In December 2021, Lisa gave a lecture at the University of Maryland to graduate students about her recovery!

My miracle baby, Lisa, is expected to make a full or very near-full physical and cognitive recovery. She is in touch with her friends daily, takes guitar lessons, works out, reads, crochets scarves for her friends, and has a plan to go to graduate school in Canada to study International Affairs so that she can be better equipped to work again with refugee children and their families who she loves so well.

THE TOOL

Dear Reader,

The story is not over. Maybe, one day I'll tell the rest of it. But I learned a lot. Perhaps some words of wisdom and guidance will be of interest and use to you. Maybe, they will help you navigate your lives.

Under the best of circumstances, living a well-lived life is complicated and difficult. It's both what we come into the world with and how we start it that gives us the seat to participate and watch things unfurl. Trust what you've been given.

There are things you can do to help you steer through the good, bad, and the difficult.

Bring your children up so they feel loved. Tell them all the time, show them all the time, whether you think they're too young to understand or not. They will. And they will appreciate it. They will develop trust in you to help them if times get tough even after they grow into adolescence!

We used to say in the 60s and 70s: question authority. Stand up and advocate for yourself and your loved ones. Speak up and speak out, be bold, take calculated risks, challenge the status quo, and forgive yourself as you make mistakes. These will help you work through the difficult beginnings and the rocks or boulders—even the avalanches along the way.

Get the information that you need in whatever manner you can. Reach out to experts and do your research.

Call on the emotional help you may need. You should neither feel alone nor are you alone. There are people to help you. Don't be afraid to get that support.

But, perhaps most of all, trust your gut—listen to your thoughts, trust what your body is telling you, listen to who you are and hold on to it because it's going to be quite a ride any way you cut it.

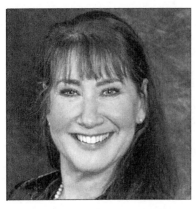

Dr. Pamela J. Pine grew up in New Jersey and has lived in Maryland since returning from a decade working overseas. She's been an international public health, development, and communication professional since the 1970s concentrating on enhancing the lives of the poor and underserved groups. Pamela has worked throughout the world from Latin America to Oceania on many difficult issues, including Hansen's Disease (leprosy), HIV, tropical diseases, childhood immunization programs, and maternal and child health. She speaks Arabic and French. Pamela is a professor of public health, an international health consultant, and the founder and director of an international program focused on preventing, treating, and mitigating child sexual abuse (CSA) and adverse childhood experiences (ACEs). She developed a comprehensive CSA/ACEs prevention/mitigation model led by local presence, adaptable for any country. She's an expert in CSA and trauma prevention/mitigation and is called upon by the media to provide authoritative input. She was honored in 2017 with a Lifetime Achievement Award in Advocacy from the Institute on Violence, Abuse, and Trauma (IVAT) in San Diego, California. Pamela is on the board of the National Partnership to End Interpersonal Violence, an advisor to IVAT, and on the Advisory Board of the Clinical and Counseling Psychology Review, Lahore, Pakistan. Pamela's Ph.D. is from UMD, her MPH from Johns Hopkins Bloomberg School of Public Health, and her International Affairs Degree from Ohio University. Given a childhood interest in art and ongoing training at Eastman School of Music and Cornell University, she continues to sing, paint, and write and is a published author. Pamela spends time with family and friends, gardens, travels, reads, and exercises in her free time.

Connect with her on the following sites:

Email: pamelajpine@gmail.com

Website: https://drpamelajpine.com

LinkedIn: https://www.linkedin.com/in/pamela-j-pine-3123b78/

CHAPTER 19

A MOTHER'S HEART SONG

LOVE NEVER FAILS OR LOSES HOPE

Pat Bell, Educator, Truth-Seeker

MY STORY

As a girl, I came to understand what is expected of a strong mother. I stood around the kitchen table with her, learning to cook, bake fresh bread and muffins, clean, and sew. I would reflect back on these moments later in life and experience the sheer exhaustion motherhood can bring. Therefore, most mothers choose a helper. "Tag, you're it! I spoke out loud in a small nostalgic whisper." Yes, I was the helper, the second hand, the one always just a few feet away.

Mother wasn't easy to know in our coming of age years, but I longed to forge a relationship with her. I observed her shortcomings wordlessly. Her mothering style directly impacted the way I would come to raise my own children. Defining life events tend to affect the mental psyche of human beings, and inevitably their behavior and response to future life events, many times without consciously knowing. I grew up in the deep south in the mid-70s and 80s, where everyone was family, blood, or otherwise. My childhood memories were of long summers, playing with friends, and being kept busy with household chores. My brother and I didn't like spending entire Saturdays doing chores. But chores were as much a part of our upbringing as eating, sleeping, and breathing.

I sometimes felt that the chores distracted me from play, and like any other child, I loathed the never-ending list. However, when I became a mother and had children of my own, it became easier for me to understand the need for a helper—the child or children who would step in on the days when the mother is overwhelmed and offers a bit of saving grace.

My mother grew up on a farm as well. Her paternal aunt and grandmother raised her. It was a hard life for her. She carried water up and down hills, worked in fields, and helped to feed the animals and milked cows. It was very hard work for a child, and I doubt she had much time to play with friends, dolls, or toys. She was named after her grandmother, Ellen.

The longer I observe human beings and life, I've come to understand that life works in circles.

My mother was not a hugger. Nor did she read us bedtime stories. Nevertheless, she fostered the love of reading in her children. There were always piles of books in the house, including dictionaries and encyclopedias. Exposure to books about faraway places and heroes and heroines intrigued a little girl growing up in the south, which gave her the ability to dream and pursue higher education.

Mother was very stern sometimes. She never accepted excuses. It was her way, or there would be consequences. But she grew up during a time when black parents weren't afforded the leisure of excuses. Life was harder back then and more restrictive. Jobs were scarce, wages were low, and poverty enveloped neighborhoods. So, my mother always expected her children to do the right things and be where they said they would be. I know she loved us. Although, that love was rarely voiced, especially in my youth.

"Does your face light up when your child walks in the room?" Toni Morrison

As a child, when life was more difficult, mother's face rarely lit up. Even so, she was a hands-on mother. Well, as much as her heart and energy would allow, as she had her day-to-day struggles managing finances, cooking, chores, and looking after three children. Trying to make ends meet with the small amount of money that my father earned from working on a farm was a daunting task.

Mother was very intelligent, but her ability to attend high school was an unrealized dream. She was too busy helping her grandmother and aunt run their farm. She dreamed of travel and wanted much more from life than she received. Consequently, the rearing of children and very little money for travel stifled those dreams. How many mothers can identify with putting the needs of the family first and burying unrealized dreams?

"Suddenly, I realize that if I stepped out of my body, I would break into blossom." A Blessing, by James Wright.

The passage of time can be a dream stealer. Mother was excellent at managing our household finances, and I would assist with household documents and paperwork. Even though we were poor, we always had the basic necessities of life. We had toys, a home, new clothes when needed, vehicles, and food on the table. My father worked very long, hard hours in order to provide for us.

My mother and I weren't friends early on. Our personalities were very different. I always led with empathy, and my mother always said exactly what she thought. Even though I was her helper, we didn't have deep conversations. However, as my mother got older and I became a mother myself, the dynamics of our relationship changed for the better. Near the end of her life, we had a loving friendship and mutual respect for one another.

My mother could drive, but she never got a driver's license due to her poor eyesight. On the days that my father was unable to drive her to the store, she and I walked to the grocery store. Living in a small town, usually, a neighbor would stop and offer us a ride. But if no one offered a ride, we just kept walking. I look back now on some of those experiences and smile. Those are memories I can't replace. Plus, many of my childhood experiences instilled a resilience I would need later in life as a divorced mother of three, and having a child who would endure a long-term illness.

I considered my mother a very strong, dominant mother figure even though she stood five feet tall. She said what she felt, and never apologized. Meanwhile, I was a very sensitive child, and her way of mothering threw me off balance. Nevertheless, I loved her but rarely voiced it. As the years quickly passed, she began to rely on my steady hand, never too far away when needed. Even when I moved away and returned home for visits with my children, I was never quite able to relinquish the role of helper. I spent my visits doing chores or styling my mother's hair. I didn't mind. I knew that someday our time together would end.

The role of helper would continue until our final earthly parting, her final breath.

I descend from a lineage of strong women. I had the privilege to be able to escape to some of these women as a child. They made life a little easier. Some even paid me to do their chores. As a very young girl, I worked next to the same aunt who reared my mother. I came to understand the face of hard work, earning your own money, and making it work for you. Even small amounts of money. *Endless green beanstalks brushed against my small thin shoulder. It tickles for a moment.* Then, my eyes focused on the brown basket, sitting on the rich soil beneath. I'm supposed to fill it with fresh beans. *I inhale deeply, then exhale, and I begin working next to my aunt. I was eight years old.*

Because my mother could be stern with us, I vowed to be more lenient when I became a mother. I would listen with a closer ear to understand. I would speak in kinder tones and assist with homework as needed. While my life hasn't been quite as hard as my mother's, there was still room for mistakes, imperfections, and, yes, the dreaded fatigue! Consequently, as we settle into motherhood, we begin to understand our own mothers better. Even mothers should be allowed some grace.

My children are allowed to have opinions and to share them. Even though there are a few chores, they never interfered with their playtime. "Mom, shoot the ball. You can't hit it from there!" When my children were younger, I always played games with them. I attempted to see them when they walked into the room. I wanted to know my children as individuals fully. I asked questions about their school day and activities. I haven't been perfect, trust me. I missed some school activities.

TO A CERTAIN CANTATRICE

"Here take this gift!
I was reserving it for some small hero, speaker, or general,
One who should serve the good old cause, the great Idea, the progress, and
freedom of the race;
Some brave comforter of despots, some daring rebel;
But I see that what I was reserving belongs to you just as much as to any."

~Walt Whitman

Doesn't every woman who has bravely taken on the role of motherhood, whether biologically or otherwise, that has done her utmost best, qualify for hero status? As Whitman states, it's not always the grandiose deed that deserves recognition and honor. But also the small daily deeds which nourish the hearts and minds of children, day after day, year after year. A mother's job is to chase out the cold and replace it with warmth. At least, on the days where exhaustion has not taken over, and she feels confident that she can bear the challenges the day may bring.

The silent warm night carried her sniffles like drifting sadness from the sky. Mother sat on the front porch in the dark summer's night, having a gut cleansing cry as most strong mothers do when they think no one else is around to hear. I wanted so much to offer her comfort. But, we still hadn't developed the closeness that would have allowed us to bond for a moment over the sadness that engulfed her. So I stood there as silently as a tiny mouse, in the dark shadows. Motherhood can sometimes feel isolating for stay-at-home mothers who choose to devote all of their time to raising their children.

Mothering is a life-altering event. We love our children. We want the best for them. But, unfortunately, mothering doesn't come with a guide. It should be instinctive and led with empathy, thoughtfulness, kindness, and love. As my mother and I grew into our roles, we became the best of friends. We learned to forgive each other's shortcomings. We shared secrets and offered listening ears and support. She became the only one I felt comfortable with crying aloud to when days were long and tedious after my divorce. She became my anchor when I felt my ship moving unsteadily. Mother learned to show empathy and listen with an understanding ear. She became my faithful confidante, and we'd speak every day, sometimes two or three times a day. We'd speak about nothing and then, everything.

"It is sheer good fortune to miss somebody before they leave you." Sula, Toni Morrison.

I missed my mother, my friend, my confidante before she left us. I often wondered what I would do without our daily chats and check-ins. I will always miss her. Even though some days, it feels like she's close enough to hear even my faintest whisper.

I loved to send mother flowers for her birthday and Mother's Day. I believe in the old adage to give flowers while a loved one lives, both literally and figuratively.

I would always send fresh flowers. I never believed in sending artificial flowers except on what would be her last birthday. Mother had arthritis, and she warned me about the work it involved to prepare the fresh flowers for their vase. So this time, I sent her a beautifully prepared arrangement of silk flowers. "I just got your flowers. These are the prettiest flowers that I've seen! Thank you! I'm going to keep them right here in the living room until you can come home and see them." She did.

The sun was barely peeking from the sky as I arrived home. "You were right, Mama. These are the prettiest silk flowers!" They were arranged in a pretty basket with a pink silk bow. The bouquet included beautiful long-stemmed hot pink Chrysanthemums. It was a good feeling to know that she enjoyed her flowers! "I told you that they were going to stay there until you could see them." As fate would have it, Mother would transition during that visit. And I, the second hand, was right next to her, gently caressing her forehead, while praying for grace and a safe arrival back to the Father.

THE TOOL

You cannot pour from an empty cup. Motherhood is not about perfection. It's about doing the best you can and seeking help and guidance when you're feeling exhausted. Stress and the inability to properly handle it is a major cause of mental and physical illness. The body and mind can function and heal when stress levels are reduced.

I encourage all mothers, new and seasoned, to practice self-care (mental and physical) as a daily ritual.

I will guide you through the relaxation and manifestation tool. Here is what you will need: Approximately 20 minutes of uninterrupted time every morning or evening, a pen and a journal, a comfortable place to lie down, a scented candle, and music. I prefer classical music.

According to Oxford Dictionary, *relaxation is when the body and mind are free from tension and anxiety.*

Manifestation is the conscious creation of circumstances and outcomes that make for a fulfilling life, according to the Berkeley Well-Being Institute.

Guidelines to consider as you practice the relaxation and manifestation activity:

1. Be gentle with yourself and your thoughts.
2. Focus on the moment you're in. It's the most important moment and the only one you have absolute control over.

Begin by lying down on the floor on a mat or in bed. Your arms should be at your sides, palms up. Before lying down, make sure that your scented candle is burning safely, and classical music is playing softly in the background. Your notebook and

pen should also be easy to access shortly after the relaxation exercise. The manifestation part of this exercise will take approximately five minutes.

Close your eyes while taking in the aroma of the room. Be kind with your thoughts and non-judgmental. You may be distracted focused on the children. But, for the next 20 minutes, focus on your healing and rejuvenation.

Now, focus on your breathing. During the breathing exercise, you will complete four repetitions. First, inhale slowly while mentally counting to four, then exhale slowly while counting to four. With each breath inhale, focus on tense areas in your body. As you exhale, focus on releasing the tension in those areas. Allow your breathing to cleanse your mind with each breath. It's okay if you lose focus for a moment. Gently refocus your attention. After the first two breathing sets, tension should begin to release.

Once your mind is relaxed, and you have completed two out of four breathing exercises, begin to think of two goals you would like to achieve for yourself and your family this year. Still paying attention to your breathing, begin to manifest the two goals that would change your family's life. As you inhale slowly to four and exhale to four, focus on your goals. Think about how wonderful it would feel to be able to have your goals manifest for your family this year.

After the last set of four breaths, lie still for a moment, with your eyes closed. Begin to listen to the noises around you, whether it's a bluejay chirping softly outside of your window or the laughter of children in the living room. Allow your heart to be fully open to this new awakened feeling of relaxation and purpose. Now, slowly open your eyes and reacquaint yourself with your environment. Next, locate the pen and journal lying nearby. Let your mind drift back to the two goals you'd like to manifest for your family this year. Clearly articulate those two goals on paper in specific detail. Write down how it will feel to achieve the goal. How will it catapult your family physically, emotionally, spiritually, financially forward?

As you practice the relaxation and manifestation exercise daily, begin to develop a vision board for your family. Put the vision board up on the wall, in the bedroom, in the kitchen, or wherever the family can see it daily. Allow all family members to add to the vision board, and when goals begin to manifest for the family, check them off. This is a proven method. Read your vision board at least once or twice a day. See yourself achieving your goals.

I have scriptures written on my vision board. "Write the vision and make it plain." Habakkuk 2:2. I believe in a higher power. I know that I can do nothing without His grace and mercy. I have scriptures concerning healing and health on my vision board and scriptures concerning abundance.

Repeat the relaxation and breathing exercises daily. Add two different goals you desire to manifest for your family every day. You may want improved health for a family member, a friend, or a closer relationship with God. You can include whatever goal you'd like in the manifestation portion of your breathing. But then remember to write the vision down in your journal and transfer the goals to your family's vision board.

As mothers, we must summon the strength and mental fortitude to continue the good work and raise God's most precious gift to us as women.

"I go forth alone and stand as ten thousand." *Our Grandmothers* by Maya Angelou

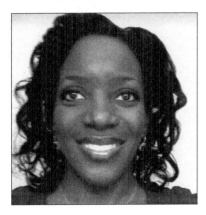

Pat Bell is an author, published poet, educator, and serial entrepreneur. Her companies are service-based. She is a Generational Wealth Mentor. She creates generational wealth as a real estate investor and stock market maven. Pat enjoys helping others free up their time to have more time to spend doing the things that they love with their families. She is currently developing an education company that intends to fill in the gap that may exist in a regular classroom setting. Pat is a published poet. Her long-time passions have been reading and writing poetry. It puts her spirit at ease while engaging her mind with delightful prose.

Pat began her career as an English as a Second Language teacher. She has taught English at her local school district and community college, and he enjoys teaching both children and adults. Consequently, her passion for entrepreneurship leads her to combine helping families, students, and business ownership.

Pat enjoys reading self-help books, riding her bike, and walking in the sunshine listening to the bird's chirp. She enjoys spending time with her magnificent family. She is a continuous life student and feels that helping herself become a better person is a journey that should never cease. Her goal is to leave the world a better place. Pat is committed to helping children and families to become all they were intended to be, as they remain true to their authentic selves and pay attention to that small divine voice within.

Connect with Pat:

On her website:

https://www.thewellnessuniverse.com/world-changers/patbabers/

https://www.amazon.com/Pat-Bell/e/B09MWNBPCW/

On LinkedIn: https://www.linkedin.com/in/pat-bell-688b3147

CHAPTER 20

MOTHERING
FROM THE GUT

WHAT TO DO WHEN THE INTERNET
DOESN'T HAVE THE ANSWER

Sally Martin

MY STORY

"Okay, so let's find our adapted warrior one pose—feel the strength in your back leg, lengthen your spine, keep your heart space broad and open. Perhaps your baby is snuggled high to one side of your heart, looking back over your shoulder. Perhaps your baby is facing forward, and you can allow them to rest on your front thigh. Maybe you will stay here a moment. Breathe. Perhaps you can release one arm and stretch your fingertips up to the sky. Here we are, strong warrior mums of Wanstead!"

I'm teaching my Baby Yoga class.

Eight women stand in a circle, in this sacred space we've created, in this tall church hall with its wooden beamed ceiling and arched leaded windows. The light sprinkles in.

"Let's walk with our babies. Feel the weight of your body and your baby with each step. Make it rhythmic."

I sing a song as the mums and their babies walk around the room.

We're walking a path, literally and metaphorically, that so many women have walked before us. It's said, and I have observed it for myself, that if you ask a group of women with babies to walk in a circle, they always walk counter-clockwise. Nobody seems to know why. There's something magical in mothering, isn't there?

"Lovely, now, slowly come to stillness."

Babies often seem to prefer movement to stillness. I know that standing still for too long probably isn't the right choice for this class, so I suggest the mums move instinctively with their baby.

"Perhaps your baby likes to be rocked side to side, bounced up and down, or swung gently forward and back."

I see the quiver of a few lips, the look of concern flicker across a few pairs of eyes. Someone finally says, "But I read that if we rock them, they'll never want to be put down."

What we read can sometimes cause us to shut down our instincts to connect and be playful with our babies.

"Just do what feels right for you and your baby at this moment. I'm going to teach Little Dips, but if it's not for you, just leave it out, do only what feels right for you and your baby."

I've observed the rhythms of new mothers that arrive in my classes. I've listened to their experiences, fears, and worries. I've noticed their pain and patterns. I've learned to guide them through the practices I teach—to let them explore the effects of positive touch and gentle movement for themselves. But I know each parent must follow their own path. I may lead the dance, but the tune is their own.

I encourage the mums to notice their own baby's cues as they bend their knees, and one, two, three, bounce their baby down an inch or two. The babies begin to settle, and the mums start to smile.

Before the session, I've practiced my routine of preparation. I know to manage the class, I need to stay centered. Over time, I've learned to relax and trust in my teaching, and in turn, my clients have relaxed and trusted in me.

The participants lift one knee and, with support, balance their baby on their thighs. We giggle together as we march around the room like soldiers. One baby starts to cry, the movement is too much for them perhaps, or maybe it's time for a feed? I've learned to accept that classes do not always go to plan—babies bring their own unpredictability, and so I know I'll likely need to change and adapt the session at some point or other.

We balance. We wobble. We balance again.

The mums chat as we sit together with steaming cups of herbal tea. Our conversations are wide and varied, but nearly always, someone raises the concerns and expectations they or others have of their parenting methods. I feel that today, everyone just wants to talk and share their troubles.

One mum sighs and says, "I wish somebody would just tell you what you're meant to do. There are so many different views and opinions that I've lost all sense of listening to what I think my baby needs."

There are nods of agreement throughout the group.

I've lost count of the number and names of books, blogs, apps, and social media groups that have fallen in and out of favor over the last 15 years amongst the new mums in my classes. Sometimes these can, of course, prove helpful; a guide or roadmap is, after all, often required when we're in new territory. But they don't always show us the right way, or *our way.*"

I try to reassure my class.

I wonder if all the noise stops us from listening to what we know all along. I believe the instinct to nurture and to mother lives inside us all. This can look different to different people. I am, after all, not a mother myself. Yet I feel drawn to facilitate these classes, which provide their own form of nurture and create a safe space to mother and be mothered.

I've learned to hold space for myself and others in teaching these sessions. I'm not teaching my clients how to parent but guiding them and enabling them (I hope) to hear their gut instincts once again. Sometimes, the only way forward is to put aside everyone else's expectations and do what feels right for you. This is how I built Buddha Baby—it wasn't planned; I just felt compelled to pursue it.

"So, how can we hear our intuition?" I ask my class.

We discuss the importance of accepting babies as they are, of relaxing in the moment, of the shared but unique experience of mothering and feeling our way forward, of trusting that it will all be okay, of letting go of expectations from others. We agree to practice this in our baby yoga sessions.

Towards the end of my class, I help the participants prepare for Savasana—relaxation time. Some babies feed, some babies sleep, and some are rhythmically walked around the room. In whatever way suits, mothers and babies snuggle together.

I've used the practice of writing, rehearsing, and repeating affirmations for many years and often draw on them in my classes. They're not for everybody, but many of my clients have told me they help and resonate with them. I choose one to sum up the session.

We try to sit in comfort, where we are.

Soft music whispers in the background, and the clock patiently ticks on the wall. After a while, the music ceases, and I bring together the Tibetan chime-bells, their resonance reaching out across the void of the hall.

From the Tao of Motherhood, by Vimala McClure, I read aloud to my class, "As the river finds the sea, you will find your way."

THE TOOL

I often draw on this process in my classes where new parents attend with their young babies. We may rehearse this at the beginning of a session to settle everyone and remind ourselves that the babies rule the class. Our role is to follow their guide. I may also encourage this practice during the main activity of the session, especially if everything goes a bit wild!

It's just five simple steps.

I hope this will help you put aside the piles of guidebooks in times of stress and allow you to trust your gut and follow the instinctive mother within you.

I've included some affirmations for you too. If these aren't useful to you, please feel free to ignore them. You can still follow the five steps: accept, relax, feel, trust, release.

STEP ONE: ACCEPT

Affirm to yourself that you accept what is happening, as it's happening. As chaotic and unpredictable as the moment is right now, or will be at some point soon, there is likely a need your baby is trying to communicate to you. This might be physical, such as hunger or a nappy change, which are perhaps relatively easy to notice and attend to. Emotional needs might be more difficult to decipher; although they can be glaring and loud, they can also be subtle and are perhaps more challenging to soothe. Perhaps there is pain or a need for sleep, which might cause angst and worry for you. Accepting that babies are complex human beings is the first step.

I often start my classes this way. It's also a great way to connect with your baby daily, or even during any moment when you don't know what else to do.

Choose one of the following:

- Hold your baby in whichever way you both find comfortable and comforting.
- Place one hand on your baby's belly and the other on your belly.
- Rest one hand on your baby's heart space and one hand over your own heart.
- Gather up your baby's arms and legs and hug them gently into their torso for a *containment hug*.

Whichever method you choose, rest your hands on or around your baby.

Gaze softly at your baby if possible, or gently close your eyes.

If your baby is vocal, let them say what it is they need to say. Listen.

Affirm:

- I accept my baby as they are in this moment.
- I listen and observe without judgment before deciding on my next action.
- I look with loving eyes.

STEP TWO: RELAX

Wherever you are with your baby, take three deep breaths.

Let your shoulders drop away from your ears. Let your arms feel heavy. Let your hands release any tension. Let your fingers relax.

Even though in a difficult moment, relaxing feels almost impossible and unlikely.

Affirm:

- I allow myself to relax with my baby.

STEP THREE: FEEL

Now tune in. Ignore all the *shoulds* and notice the *feels*. Ask yourself what *feels* like the right thing to do at this moment. Not what your mum or mother-in-law says you should do. Not what your friend who has three kids already says you should do. Not what that book or blog post said you should do. Instead, what you feel somewhere deep down within your belly, heart, and soul is the right thing to do for you and your baby.

Ask yourself, what is my baby asking of me at this moment?

What you choose to do, the next action you take, probably won't even be a conscious, cognitive thing. It will be something so instinctive that you're moved to do it without thinking too hard. Don't panic. You don't have to do it for life, just for this moment.

Affirm:

- When I don't know what to do next, I ask, what feels right for us at this moment?
- We are flexible and free; we go with the flow.
- I allow my baby to be my teacher; I follow their lead.

Then, you feel it out. Whatever action it is you have chosen, try it out. Notice your baby's reactions. Notice how you feel. It may be a bit uncomfortable at first but give it a few minutes; not all reactions are immediate.

STEP FOUR: TRUST

Keep going! If, after a few minutes, it seems to be working, don't stop. It may take a few minutes, as not all positive reactions are instant, and babies need time to adjust. Observe, then continue, or adapt if you need to.

Trust that you can change the action you have chosen at any time. Try something else if you need to, but don't rush, switching from one thing to the next too quickly; this is likely to overwhelm and confuse your baby, wear you out, and make you feel the situation is hopeless. Just stick with what you're doing, accept the moment, keep breathing, keep relaxing, keep *feeling* it out.

That's your intuition. That's your gut instinct right there. When things start to settle, there is nothing else to do but continue to follow this path. The ancient mothering lineage deep within us kicks in. Allow yourself to continue to do what feels right. After all, it's working. You knew all along. You knew within your gut that this was what you and your baby needed to do. It's just that it got noisy out there, so we forgot to hear, and we forgot how to listen.

Affirm:

- I trust my intuition. I follow what feels right for my baby and me.
- I permit myself to follow what feels right for us.
- I know we will find our way.

STEP FIVE: RELEASE

Finally, be grateful. You managed the moment. There is, if only for a short while, peace. A lull in the chaos. A moment to reflect. Maybe only now can you feel the love? Perhaps only now can you allow your shoulders to drop away from your ears, your arms to feel heavy, your hands to release tension, and your fingers to relax. Take three deep breaths.

There is no one right way, there is only your way, and you found it. Let everyone else find their way. It's not your job to teach them, only to hand down those skills to your children, modeling through your practice. You can take the lessons you've learned and release those teachings that don't resonate with you.

Affirm:

- I appreciate this moment with my baby.
- I am not held back by illusions of how things should be.
- Everything is happening perfectly, in the right way, and at the right time for us.
- I lovingly release others to their own lessons.

In that short moment, you switched off the noise and got back to listening to your gut instinct. You attended to your well-being and your baby's well-being. You did not force or push; you felt your way through. You're deeply connected with the millions of mothers who have mothered before, whatever form it took.

Earlier in this chapter, I quoted from the *Tao of Motherhood* by Vimala McClure; I return to that now. She says, "Knowing how things work is helpful to you. But remember, mothers have mothered since the dawn of time, and it all seems to work out in the end."

This will be true for you too, for you, too, are a strong mother.

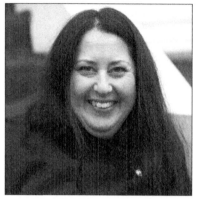

Sally Martin is the founder and creative director of Buddha Baby. With over 20 years of experience in education, Sally combines her passion for teaching with her interest in holistic well-being practices. Sally is a consultant in primary PSHE education and babywearing, baby massage, baby yoga, massage-in-schools instructor, massage therapist, and yoga enthusiast.

Sally facilitates classes for new parents and their babies in her local area, East London, UK. She teaches traditional parenting skills, promotes human connection, gentle sensory stimulation, and mindful movement. She offers pregnancy and well-woman massage from the sanctuary of her beautiful home, where she also works as an educational resource writer.

Sally loves baking for her classes in her little pink kitchen, with the door swung open to the garden and the radio on. She also loves anywhere a bit wild and windy, ancient stories of goddesses, a good cup of tea, elephants, and seahorses.

Connect with her on the following sites:

Website: www.buddhababywanstead.co.uk

Facebook: www.facebook.com/buddhababylondon

Instagram: www.instagram.com/buddhababylondon

LinkedIn: www.linkedin.com/in/sallymartineducation

CLOSING CHAPTER

Christina Morris

Eyes open. Eyes closed. Drifting in and out. For me, the upside to pregnancy insomnia and vivid dreams was that big life dreams happened—chemical messages pumping through my blood. Ideas came, and the ultimate feeling of flow radiated through my body. A buzzing feeling made me spring from my bed in the early hours, head to my office, and scribble in my notepad until my wrist and the side of my palm hurt from pressing passionately into the pen and down onto the page. The idea for this book came to me then. I was inspired and invigorated by becoming a mother.

I'm a true believer that everything happens for a reason, and over the course of my pregnancy and in early motherhood, I was lucky enough to cross paths with the ladies in this book. I know they were drawn to me, and I to them for a reason.

My dream is to create the book that I wish existed for me with voices of women who have lived and walked their motherhood journey. Although each journey is unique, there is no doubt that you can learn a special tool from each of these mothers that will work for you and your situation.

If we're able to help one mother even slightly, then we will have fulfilled the purpose of this book. This book is powerful. It's made with so much love, and these ladies have poured their heart and soul onto the page, as have I.

If you're reading this and you're struggling, or you have struggled, know this, you are not just a survivor; you are a thriver!

ACKNOWLEDGMENTS

Thank you to friends and family who read early copies.

To my husband for always listening to me reading my work aloud and for being patient and encouraging. Thank you for the love you so easily give me and the pure love we share with our son.

Thank you to my mum, dad, sisters, wider family, and Morris family for always being happy for me and supporting my ideas and aspirations. I love you all dearly.

My great friends Laura Mc and Lucy for proofreading so many things during and since university—such reliable, kind friends.

My oldest friends: Sarah, Rachel, Anna, Laura, and Jenny. Your friendship is a joy. Thank you for your support.

Ebony: I'm so glad I met you. You are so caring and talented in everything you do. Thank you for your continued support.

Chuck and Naomi: You are inspiring. Thank you for your encouragement and help.

Thank you, Laura Di Franco and your team, for believing in this vision and bringing me into the Brave Healer Productions world. It is amazing, and I have met such wonderful people. Laura, you are a force of nature and a kind heart. It has been a joy attending your course, your webinars, and learning more about being a brave businesswoman. I look forward to learning even more from you.

An enormous gargantuan, thank you to wonderful authors who have made this book possible. Working with you and reading your stories has been awe-inspiring. I'm so glad to have met you, and without you, this dream wouldn't have been possible.

To the readers, I have an abundance of gratitude for you. Thank you from deep in my soul for choosing this book.

To the past version of me, you did it. You pulled through the abyss of overwhelm and so much more. The scared, self-doubting mother you think you are now will soon be proud of the strong mother you actually are.

Thank you, Universe.

"Christina is one of those rare people with the perfect mix of sensitivity and fierceness. She has an enormous heart that is always open. Her kind, caring nature makes her a truly wonderful friend but, more importantly, a great mother, and when she needs it, her fierceness kicks in, and she can move mountains."

Jo Behari, Author, Entrepreneur, DIY expert, and TV presenter

"Christina is a determined person. Always happy to embrace new challenges. She likes to enjoy whatever she does. For me, it's been a pleasure to see her going from pregnancy to motherhood in such a natural way. This is something that I believe is a basic need to keep your mental health intact as a parent, and this will, of course, go back to the child. I am looking forward to reading Strong Mothers to see what Christina has to share with all of us."

Maria Carrera, Master Sensei, Business Owner of Carrera's Studio and Co-Author of *Black Belt Women*

"Christina radiates kindness and has the rare gift of making anyone and everyone feel heard and understood. Beautiful, inspiring, and intelligent, her energy is contagious."

Kelly Southcott, Entrepreneur of Kivo Transformation - Digital Transformation & Coaching

COACHING FOR PARENTS-TO-BE

I have years of experience in coaching, but since becoming a mother, coaching mums-to-be has been my passion. Are you feeling overwhelmed? Do you want to be successful without feeling swamped? Talk to me.

I transform the experience of ambitious mamas-to-be with positive actions and prioritization with healing research and expertise. I will guide you through my principles and help you overcome hurdles to live a healthy, empowered life.

https://www.yes-mindset.com/contact

HIRE CHRISTINA TO SPEAK
AT YOUR NEXT EVENT

Book Christina for speaking events to show that you value potential parents, parents-to-be, and new parents and genuinely care about their healthy mindset at your business or organization. She will dispel their trepidation and work with you to ensure parents-to-be are supported.

Christina has appeared on podcasts and is happy to discuss all things motherhood and/or mindset on your podcast.

yesmamamindset@gmail.com

ANOTHER BOOK WITH CHRISTINA

Read *Black Belt Women, Lessons on Perseverance*. This book is full of amazing women achieving martial arts accomplishments against all odds.

Christina's chapter:

Chapter 10

No Excuses

https://www.yes-mindset.com/product-page/black-belt-women-lessons-on-perseverance

Printed in Great Britain
by Amazon